C000258026

**EACH BOOK SOLD
FEEDS A HUNGRY CHILD
FOR A MONTH**

BANANA MAN

The inspirational story of how one man's mission to help a child led him to become an accidental hero to thousands more

KEVIN ALLEN

Banana Man
by Kevin Allen

Book Design and Setting by
Neil Coe (neil@cartadesign.co.uk)

Set in Goudy 11.5 on 18pt

First published in 2007.
Second edition in 2010 by;

Ecademy Press
6 Woodland Rise, Penryn, Cornwall UK TR10 8QD
info@ecademy-press.com
www.ecademy-press.com

Printed and Bound by;
Lightning Source in the UK and USA

Printed on acid-free paper from managed forests. This book is printed on demand, so no copies will be remaindered or pulped.

ISBN-978-1-905823-73-4

The right of Kevin Allen to be identified as the author of this work has been asserted in accordance with sections 77 and 78 of the Copyright Designs and Patents Act 1988.

A CIP catalogue record for this book is available from the British Library.

All rights reserved. No part of this publication may be reproduced in any material form (including photocopying or storing in any medium by electronic means and whether or not transiently or incidentally to some other use of this publication) without the written permission of the copyright holder except in accordance with the provisions of the Copyright, Designs and Patents Act 1988. Applications for the Copyright holders written permission to reproduce any part of this publication should be addressed to the publishers.

Dedicated to

The mighty Zulu nation

and the forgotten children of Zululand

"Zulu" means children of God

Contents

Foreword

22nd **January 1879**

It was eerily quiet as Corporal William Allen and Private John Williams gazed to the hills anxiously. Moments later and a low chugging beat of a train could be heard in the distance.

But it wasn't a train; it was thousands of Zulus marching to war in defence of their kingdom. Fear built amongst the handful of soldiers, as the sound beat in their ears with an ever increasing intensity. Then from the hillside a swamp of Zulus charged. "Here they come!" cried Sergeant Henry Gallagher. "As thick as grass and as black as thunder." William stared at John, both men fearing they were about to die a bloody death.

They didn't know then that this battle would go down as legend, or that they were about to change the course of history for an entire nation.

Nor could they know that their actions this day would ripple through time, changing the destiny of an ordinary, unassuming family man from England, 126 years later...

What a difference a day makes

As the passenger behind me stood up and brushed past me, I woke from my light sleep. I'd only been asleep for a short time, but it was always the same on the overnight flight to Johannesburg, and I dreaded it each time I left home.

I rubbed my tired eyes and looked for the time. It was 4:44 a.m. and I laughed as the numbers flashed in front of me. "Of course it is" I said to myself, knowing that the next few days were going to be as mysteriously magical as my previous adventures in Africa.

What an amazing few years it had been, I thought to myself as I shifted uncomfortably in my seat. I rummaged through my backpack and found the photos I'd brought to show my old friend, Hedwig. As I stared at them silently, I smiled, remembering the incredible and bizarre events which had occurred over the last four years, and how it had all begun one wintry night in February.

February 26th 2005

It had been a cold, blustery Saturday night, and a time to relax and recuperate after a long week of work. But then life hadn't been particularly relaxing for me lately.

I'd lost a business a few years earlier, which had been accompanied by an unpleasant mountain of debt. Money had been tight for a long time, and had been causing financial frustration and numerous personal pressures within my family.

Tonight however was peaceful. My wife, Joanne, had taken our children to see their grandparents and I was enjoying the relative quiet of having the house to myself.

I rarely found time to watch TV, but as I sat to eat a meal, a documentary came on, highlighting the terrible plight of AIDS orphans in Zululand, South Africa.

Normally I would turn over, as I find this type of programme depressing, but the TV remote was the other side of the room and I couldn't be bothered getting up to switch channels. So in an act of lazy apathy, I sat and watched.

I had no idea, then, that my life was about to change beyond my imagination.

It wasn't long before I witnessed an impoverished and dying mother desperately trying to support thirteen children, many of whom she had taken in after they had been orphaned. She had just found out that one of her young daughters might have AIDS herself and was showing early signs of sickness. Her husband had already died of AIDS and she was scared that when she died, she would leave many young children behind to a terrible fate.

Next, a young boy's life was shattered as he watched his 38 year-old father die of AIDS in front of his eyes. He had to walk miles back in the dark to a filthy mud hut with no running water, gas or electricity. Distraught, afraid and starving, he soon broke down in tears – and so did I. His mother had already died of AIDS, a year earlier, and his brave young sister tried to comfort him in vain.

Tears were pouring down my cheeks by now and I felt nauseated, knowing that the young Zulu boy, named only as Sne, might soon be dead.

The programme continued, and so did the scenes of inhumanity.

I'm not religious and don't go to church, yet found myself looking to the heavens and angrily asking why the world allowed these horrors to happen.

A voice in my head said – "Why do you?"

I knew from that instant I would not.

Six days later I was standing in Zululand, searching for Sne and the other families I'd seen on TV just days earlier.

Every journey starts with a first step

The Journey Within

The programme had long finished by the time Joanne returned home, but as she entered the house she looked into my eyes and knew something was very wrong.

My body was on fire with an uncontrollable emotion which was overwhelming me - love, grief, rage, pain - all coursing through my veins, mixed in an unfamiliar pot of confusion and anger.

Every tiny little cell in my body was screaming at me to find the young Zulu boy, and help him, but I was battling against a mountain of inhibitions which were restricting me to the point of paralysis.

I couldn't think, I couldn't speak, I couldn't breathe...and I couldn't tell Joanne that I had to leave home to find a young African boy who needed my help.

It was ridiculous even to think I could embark on such a journey.

I left the room and tried to avoid conversation with her for the rest of the evening, as my mind was consumed with confusing thoughts of what I should do.

That night I didn't sleep, not even a wink. I was experiencing an emotional rollercoaster ride of indescribable intensity. It was as if it were my own son who was lost far away in Africa, dying and afraid.

Even more than that, it was as if it was me.

I've no idea why, but somehow I had connected with this young boy's plight and felt his fear and despair; his pain was mine now and it wasn't going to go away.

In the morning I was still fighting my deeply rooted inhibitions. I felt sick to the stomach still, and couldn't eat or drink; worse still, I couldn't look my children in the eyes knowing that a young boy might otherwise die if I did not act.

By now Joanne was becoming concerned by my agitated behaviour. She had never seen me so upset before and wanted to know what the hell was going on.

I tried to explain to her about the programme I had watched, but quickly broke down. I told her there was a young boy who desperately needed help – but he was in Africa and I did not know where he was or how I could find him.

As I spoke I knew the words sounded crazy. Joanne just held me for a brief moment then said "Go and find him".

And in that moment, she set me free.

The hardest part of my journey was over. Bursting through the inhibition to just get up and go had been extremely difficult. In no small part because I lived in a small terraced house in a deprived area of Merseyside, and my family's life savings totalled little more than £1,500.

Our street had been plagued with drug dealers, drunks and aggressive gangs of louts for the past year and we had been made virtual prisoners in our home lately.

Now I had to leave my family, friends and work all behind - and I could not explain to anyone why.

Actions speak louder than words

Accidental Coincidences?

It was less than 24 hours after I had first seen the documentary, when an incredible sequence of events started to occur.

Desperate to travel to Africa that day, I rang various travel agents, but to my dismay I found that a return ticket to Durban - a round trip involving six planes in total - could cost as much as my meagre savings of £1,500 at this short notice.

My journey was ending before it had even started.

Luckily, by coincidence, I had been introduced to a travel agent a few weeks earlier by a business contact, and he had said if I ever needed a cheap holiday to contact him and he would find me a great deal.

I quickly tracked down his phone number and called his shop, and spoke with his daughter, who was working that day. She took the details and made various calls until finally she found a flight leaving in three days' time and costing just over £800.

I wanted to leave right away, but I couldn't. In three days' time it would be.

The trouble was, if I wanted to guarantee the ticket I would have to secure it now by credit card. A few years earlier my business had collapsed and this had a negative impact on my credit history.

Frustration poured in. I didn't have a credit card and couldn't secure my ticket.

Yet, unbeknownst to me then, the fact I didn't own a credit card would save my life before the week was out!

I slept soundly that evening, partially through intense tiredness and partially through an unusual and growing feeling of contentment.

The next day I was up early and withdrew our family savings from the bank, before securing my ticket. With the balance I headed to town to buy as many supplies as I could fit into my suitcase, before converting the remaining money into South African Rand for my trip ahead.

I reached town and, incredibly, the first shop I entered was selling children's clothes at 25p per garment! I couldn't believe my luck, and picked up as many clothes as I could carry – then went back for more, then more again. The lady at the till was unimpressed with my decision to clear the shop's shelves of clothes, and thought I was buying them to resell on eBay at a profit!

She looked at me coldly, then called the shop manager, who proceeded to rant at the assistant because the clothes had been mis-priced and should have been discounted from £4.95 to £2.25 an item, not to 25p! The manager looked at the giant pile of clothes I had assembled at the till and stared at me harshly, "I'm sorry, but I can't sell you all those clothes at this price. You can purchase one top for 25p before we re-price them properly."

"But I need these clothes for orphans in South Africa," I explained, upset and disappointed. An elderly lady standing behind me in the queue started talking, "I used to live in South Africa as a child," she said, and proceeded to answer questions that had been playing on my mind about my journey, even though I didn't ask her a single question!

Then she turned sharply to the shop manager, "Once marked and displayed at this price, you have to sell these clothes to this young man under law." The manager paused for a moment, then reluctantly agreed and I soon left the shop in delight. I had just bought 80 garments of children's clothing worth around £400, having paid just £20.

Weighed down with the huge bags of cheap clothes I had just bought, I soon had to pause for breath and looked in the window of another shop. "Massive Sale" said a sign in big red letters, and I noticed that they were selling children's socks and underwear cheaply, so I struggled into the shop keenly hunting my second bargain of the day.

I picked up a huge mix of cheap underwear packs and went to the till, where two ladies were looking at me menacingly. Instantly I became self-conscious and started to turn bright red. I was buying over a hundred pairs of boys' and girls' underwear of various sizes and realised this looked pretty weird for a man in his thirties!

I looked back at the cashiers, desperate to ease my embarrassment, and explained, "I'm flying to South Africa and taking clothes to orphaned children there." The cashiers' mood changed instantly and I relaxed a little. As they bagged up the clothes they chatted with me until a lady behind me who had been listening said, "I come from Durban" – and immediately started telling me about the terrible social problems in South Africa – again answering many of the questions swirling around my mind.

This was the second South African that I had spoken to within 10 minutes, and probably only the second South African I had ever spoken with in my entire life! A timely coincidence and a much welcomed one.

By now I was delighted. I had my ticket to fly to Africa, I had met two helpful South Africans and I had bought more clothes than I could physically carry for less than £30!

I was weighed down and rapidly becoming tired, but still needed to pick up some currency before I headed home.

I soon reached a high street travel agent and stumbled through the doors, again feeling embarrassed as the staff stared at me with the mountain of bags I was carrying. I went to the cashier's desk only too aware that four pairs of eyes were following me. Shyly smiling at the cashier, I sheepishly explained I was travelling to South Africa and was taking the clothes to orphans there. He smiled back and said "You'll be needing Rand then, but I don't think I have any left - let me look."

He came back and apologised, "I only have 5,000 Rand (about £500) but it's all in ten and twenty Rand notes." I didn't understand why he was so sorry, but agreed to take the lot.

Twenty minutes later as he was still counting the hundreds of notes, I realised why he was sorry! A ten Rand note was worth less than a pound. As I saw him count out the hundreds of notes, piling them one on top of the other, I quickly visualised the size of the giant cash pile I would soon be handed.

Inadvertently, this was the exact value of currency I would need for the journey ahead. I hadn't realised then, but I would be leaving the UK feeling poor having only a few hundred pounds in my pocket – only to enter Zululand with the same amount of cash, but as a rich man, as it magically transformed into an absolute fortune in their third-world economy.

As the cashier continued to count, an ever-growing, grumbling queue was developing behind me and I began to become self-conscious again. A voice from behind piped up and said, "You're going to South Africa with that Rand, hey – that's where I am from." I must have looked puzzled as I turned to face him. This was the third South African who had introduced himself to me within half an hour and the coincidences of the day were growing bizarre. For the next few minutes the man reminisced about his time in Durban, imparting valuable information and advice about my trip ahead.

As the cashier wearily finished counting out the huge pile of Rand, I looked at him blankly and said "I'm going to need a bigger wallet." "Yes," he replied, smiling.

Weighed down with bag after bag of clothing, and with wads of money stuffed in every pocket, I slowly waddled out of town, laughing like a child, to the bemusement of onlookers.

Coincidences are opportunities in disguise

Destination Durban

Each of the next three days seemed like the passing of a month. Time had all but stopped and I desperately wanted to leave for Africa. The emotional intensity that had overwhelmed me a few days earlier was rapidly turning into frustrated anger – and my family were beginning to bear the brunt of it.

Mood swings and shortness of temper were matched by a growing feeling that the day-to-day problems of family life were trivial.

Lost school books, buses that didn't turn up on time, petty arguments over which TV channel to watch: they just didn't matter to me any more, and I was becoming increasingly distant to the world around me.

My family's experience of those few days was of course very different. The days went all too quickly for Joanne, who was by now having second (third and fourth) thoughts about me leaving for Africa; for her, day-to-day life would have added pressures and stresses whilst I was away.

My leaving home so quickly for Africa was affecting my children too.

James was only five and simply didn't want me to leave him; after a few days he gave me some of his favourite toys and told me in a way only a child can, to give them to "the poor children." I loved him so much, and didn't want to leave him, but I knew I must. I had to find the young Zulu boy named Sne and help him.

Rebecca was older; she was ten, and understood there was an element of uncertainty to the journey I was embarking on. I knew she was upset, but she was trying hard not to show it.

This was adding a lot of pressure to me and by now I was questioning what on earth I was doing. Was I right to leave my young family behind, taking all the money we had in the world, to go on a journey into the unknown – to find a boy I had never met, without any certainty of finding him, or knowing what on earth I would do if I did?

My inhibitions were trying to creep back in and exploit my fears - but the decision had been made by the heart, not by the mind, and I would stop for nothing.

The day of travel finally arrived. Joanne was crying as she helped me pack my case full of children's clothes, toys and medicines; but my thoughts were to find Sne, and help him.

Normally I detested travelling. It was almost a mini-phobia, developed from a number of near-fatal car accidents I had been involved in over the years. I especially hated driving long distances, and I loathed flying even more.

Today, however, I didn't care. I had booked a taxi to Manchester airport for my first flight to Paris, and as we drove I realised that I didn't have a clue where I was going. Yet I was filled with an incredible intensity of purpose, mixed with uncertainty and an uneasy apprehension.

Snow was falling as we drove, but I hardly noticed it. My thoughts were somewhere else. As we reached the airport there was an unusually heavy security presence – five years ago we had entered a new phase of inhuman intolerance, an age of terror where men would blow themselves up in the name of God, whilst others waged war for oil, money and power.

As I entered the airport armed police were on patrol everywhere. It suddenly dawned on me I had a suitcase full of children's clothes, medicines, toys and sweets. I wasn't exactly your normal tourist and didn't know how I was going to explain I was on a mission to find a young orphan, who I had never met, if I was searched or questioned.

I passed through the various security points with a false air of guilt and crimson red with embarrassment, but continued unchallenged, before entering the airport lounge, where I waited in patient reflection for the call to my departure gate.

A call that did not come!

Snow was falling heavily now, and whilst my mind had been elsewhere, flight after flight had been cancelled – including mine. This was disastrous; I had two connecting flights to catch, and no leeway for delays.

I was stranded in Manchester Airport, and missing my connection from Paris to Johannesburg would mean I would be delayed by at least 24 hours – a time which might prove vital in my search for Sne.

By now the runways had ground to a complete halt. Nothing was flying in or out of the airport and my mission was falling to pieces before I had even left the UK.

The hours passed, but the snow storm did not. "Why did this have to happen today of all days?" I grunted to myself angrily. As frustration built, I found a quiet corner at the end of the departure lounge to stew in private.

Deep into the night, the snow finally stopped falling and I had long lost all chance of making my first connecting flight. Finally a flight to Paris was called – and I was on it. I reluctantly made my way to the gate and boarded the plane, before sinking into my seat, feeling defeated by fate.

I arrived in Paris in the dead of night as the airport was about to close. Snow was falling heavily here too and I went to a reception point to arrange an onward flight to Johannesburg. But the next flight wouldn't leave until 11 p.m. the following day! My heart dropped as my journey began to disintegrate again.

There was nothing I could do. The receptionist told me I would be put up in a hotel for the night in Paris and should return tomorrow evening for the flight. She sent me outside and said she would send a mini-bus to transport me to the hotel in a few minutes' time.

I left the airport and stood at the roadside, but the mini-bus did not come…

Having expected to be halfway to Africa by now, I was stranded in Paris in the early hours of the morning, freezing in a pair of shorts and a t-shirt, and standing in a snowstorm.

I had plenty of South African Rand but not a single euro - and no luggage, which the airline had kept. The airport had shut, the receptionist had left. As I stood in the cold I burst out laughing – cursing the gods, asking them if they were amused at my stupidity. I was trying to save a child's life, yet I couldn't even save myself!

Time passed, and my mind was frantically thinking what to do next before I froze. Then, out of the blue, a French-Jewish taxi driver arrived at the closed airport and asked where I was heading (in English, thankfully). I explained I was stranded and told him I had no euros but needed to get to a hotel for the night and passed him the name.

He offered to take me to the hotel and seemed unconcerned that I could not pay him. He was obviously kind, but a little eccentric too. He talked the whole journey about his family, chatting happily one minute, then mumbling in complaint the next, asking then answering his own questions as he drove. His conversation was welcome, but he seemed to be distracting himself, and I'm sure at times he was more lost than me.

We eventually found the hotel and I thanked him for his kind help. He responded in a confusing mixture of French / Yiddish and drove away into the night.

I entered the welcome warmth of the hotel and thought about how, having been held up from travelling for three days in the UK, I was now going to waste another precious day in Paris.

After a short, uncomfortable sleep, I woke in the morning to my four-star surroundings. Fine foods, free drinks, luxurious accommodation, polite staff. I had not travelled for this – and wanted to get out of Paris fast.

The hours passed agonisingly slowly, and my frustration built and built, until eventually it was time to return to the airport for my next flight.

Winter snow was still falling heavily, and I wondered if I was ever going to get to Africa. I arrived at the airport to chaotic scenes of mayhem: cancelled flights, further delays and more confusion. Hours later, I finally boarded a plane.

We sat on the snow-covered runway for what seemed like an eternity. The weather had started to deteriorate again and I watched impatiently as the plane's frozen wings were de-iced.

I had left home over a day ago, but had flown little over an hour in that time, and was just about to explode with frustration when the plane's engines finally fired into life.

At long last we were in the air – and I was on my way to Africa and a destination unknown.

The long-haul flight was physically and mentally tiring, not to mention acutely uncomfortable. It was an overnight flight, but I couldn't sleep and there was little else I could do now but sit back and wait.

I started to watch one of the in-flight movies to kill some time. Ironically, the first film aired was "Constantine", a sci-fi horror film depicting the battle between good and evil. I don't much like horror films, yet I watched it, not knowing that I would soon be walking into hell myself very soon.

In the morning the long, tedious flight was finally coming to an end and as we descended rapidly towards Johannesburg airport I gained my first glimpse of the inequality that (mis)shapes South Africa.

Looking out of the plane window I saw hundreds of luxurious detached homes – each of unique design with swimming pool, sitting on large plots of private land. Right next to these fabulous homes was a massive shantytown of unimaginable poverty and squalor. This bizarre sight summed up a country engulfed in crime, corruption and self-created social problems.

I was very tired, and trying hard to comprehend the sight I had witnessed as we had landed. But my journey was far from over. So I wearily set off to reorganise my final connecting plane to Durban, knowing that my schedule was completely in tatters now.

The freezing snowstorms of Europe were long behind me now, and as I walked out to board my final flight to Durban, the African heat hit me and I felt warmth and contentment for the first time in days.

Thankfully, the flight from Johannesburg to Durban took little more than an hour, and passed without incident.

Then, after three gruelling flights, I landed at my intended destination, Durban.

And my stomach knotted, as the immensity of the task ahead hit me like a brick.

A rolling stone gathers no moss

A Driving Destiny

Standing to collect my luggage, I realised I had absolutely no idea what to do next. All I had was the name of a young Zulu boy, Sne, and the name of a Catholic nun, Sister Hedwig, who had been named on the documentary and who lived in a town called Nkandla, helping the sick and caring for the thousands of children left behind by the AIDS pandemic. I had nothing else to go on but instinct, and decided my best chance of finding Sne was to track down Sister Hedwig's convent first.

I found a tourist information centre, obtained a map of South Africa, and found Nkandla – it was hundreds of miles away, and because of the delays I had only   two days before I had to fly back home.

I asked the receptionist at the desk the best route into Nkandla, and he shook his head in disbelief. "You can't travel there from here by car," he said, "and I don't know any other form of transport you can take to get you there either. Besides, it's dangerous and no place for tourists." As he spoke, his voice held an air of concern I hadn't expected. I looked at him solemnly, "If it's dangerous for me, how safe can it be for the children left orphaned there?" He looked at me blankly, but didn't reply.

I had no choice and decided my only way into Nkandla was to hire a car. Outside the airport I found a car rental outlet, but was quickly refused a car as, again, I did not have a credit card.

I felt stranded now; for the second time in a week I had needed a credit card and felt belittled for not owning one. Feelings of dejection were overtaking me and I was rapidly reaching the point of abandoning my mission, which was now running well behind schedule.

My mind wandered for a minute, trying to assess the situation. I thought of sitting out the next two days in the comfort of Durban, perhaps finding a church or charity to hand my case of children's clothes to, before relaxing on Durban's beautiful golden beach, lapped by the warm Indian Ocean.

Having journeyed this far, my inhibitions were still trying to shackle me down, but I refused to stop, and shook them off angrily.

Sne's plight had affected me deeply and, thinking of him once more, I vowed to continue and try and find him.

I had been in Durban for less than an hour, but an overwhelming feeling of pending danger and death was beginning to grow in my gut. Despite my lack of religion I found myself arguing with God for the third time in a week, telling him I would not die on this journey, that I would return home safely to my family and that if he wanted my blood he would have to wait for another day! This feeling was to grow and grow, and I would battle with it constantly for the next few days.

My options were limited now. I could take a 5-hour or so taxi ride into Zululand – or I could not go there at all.

There was a private taxi rank outside the airport and I made my way to the first taxi waiting, which was a brand new Mercedes Benz, driven by a white South African.

I asked the driver if he could take me to Nkandla in Natal – he looked at me in surprise before saying bluntly "No". The next taxi was also a Mercedes Benz and I asked the driver if he would take me, but he quickly refused and waved me away.

The next car was a battered old wreck, and I saw the large black taxi driver looking at me eagerly, ready to snare his next tourist fare. Past his car were more gleaming Mercedes, and I tried to by-pass him to another vehicle.

He quickly cut me off and asked where I was going, "Nkandla," I said, thinking he would not take the journey. At first he paused to think, then, with a large friendly smile replied, "I do not know the way, but I will take you there safely." Glancing at his car again, I doubted this greatly.

Unfortunately, David, my Zulu cab driver, really didn't know the way.

Taking a taxi from Durban into Zululand is a bit like landing in Heathrow Airport in London, and asking a taxi driver to help you find a convent in Scotland, without having anything more than a nun's name to go on!

David knew only that Nkandla was far away, off the beaten track, across dangerous and rugged terrain – and he would soon be proved right.

After some debate we planned the best route and agreed a fare.

We drove for hours along the beautiful South African coast, before the roads slowly turned to tracks; and as the tarmac ended, so did the running water, the electricity, proper housing, access to food and healthcare and, worst of all, hope.

We were heading deep inland through beautiful dense forests and up into mountains, then down into valleys. As we travelled we talked as if we were old friends who had met again after a long absence. Like me, David was in his early thirties and married, and he had a baby daughter. His dream was to run his own taxi firm to earn a fair living, and to own his own home.

But he could not.

He was black and owned nothing of value, which meant he could not get a mortgage or even a loan to buy a better vehicle to start his own taxi firm. Apartheid should have ended in the eighties – for some it had, but for many Zulus on the bottom rung of the ladder, I'm not sure it had.

Indeed, for those out of sight of the main cities, it had probably intensified with the onslaught of an AIDS pandemic which was decimating communities as the rest of the world turned a blind eye.

As we drove deeper into rural Natal, David kept stopping at roadside stalls, encouraging me to buy fruit as he knew the local traders desperately needed the tourist Rand. The fruit only costs pennies – but the people needed the money so badly I bought bag after bag of bananas.

Before long, the taxi was full of hundreds of bananas, so we started to give the fruit out to the hungry children we passed on the roadside. David started laughing, calling me "Banana Man", a name which would later stick!

We had been driving for about four hours and the roads were deteriorating as I realised David's battered taxi was feeling the strain. We joked that if the car broke down I would have to push it up the mountain. But we knew that if it did, we would both be in real danger, as we were now many miles away from civilisation and darkness was beginning to fall.

As twilight fell, David said we should head back to the safety of the coastal road and Durban. I knew he was right, but I couldn't give up now, having come so far. I convinced him I desperately needed to reach Nkandla town – and reluctantly he agreed to continue.

Apart from the danger of being stranded in the bush, driving at night was not safe at all. David explained crime was high due to extreme poverty and that gangs would put obstacles on the road to cause car crashes, so that they could rob the occupants.

It was soon dark and it wasn't long before we saw small gangs of men within the shadows, and apprehension started to turn to fear. We were soon driving in the pitch black – out here there was nothing – no lights, no traffic, no shops. The only light we had was coming from the taxi's weak highlights. The roads were narrow and winding, with potholes and blind corners everywhere.

Occasional flashes from the headlights revealed shadowy silhouettes in the darkness. David would slow down carefully, checking the road for obstructions, before speeding up to pass quickly.

As we continued, the menace increased as we saw sporadic groups of men wandering in the darkness with large sticks and other threatening weapons. David was growing increasingly anxious, and matters got worse as we realised we were completely lost.

It was coming to the end of the summer and we could see a huge thunderstorm ahead, approaching us fast. As giant lightning bolts lit up the dark night sky David confessed thunder was a childhood fear – and he was beginning to panic.

We turned the car around and slowly retraced our steps until we found ourselves back at a small junction we had previously missed. Then, travelling another 48 kilometres along treacherous roads, we finally reached Nkandla town to our great relief.

But this relief was soon to pass.

It was late now, and Nkandla town at night was no place for a lost tourist.

I felt like we had just driven into a lawless wild-west town of old, late at night. The men who were out, were out for trouble and acting erratically, obviously high on drugs, and carrying weapons for protection or aggression.

David explained that marijuana grew naturally in the area and that the men here smoked it for 'health' benefits or to help them cope with the trauma of life. Panic was setting in by now and I did not know where to go next. There were no hotels here; no lodging or safe places of refuge.

What's more, David had completed his fare and was saying he wanted to go back home to the safety of Durban – and asking where I wanted him to drop me off in this hell-hole!

In the distance we could see something which we had not seen in many hours: lights. They were coming from a large building, and a sign pointing a little further up the road said 'Nkandla Hospital'.

That was it: the hospital would be a safe place for me to head.

As we slowly approached the hospital, it looked more like a prison in the darkness. It was surrounded by high security fences and barbed wire. David explained that the hospital was a place of food, medicines and drugs, blankets and beds – all luxury items for the impoverished Zulus of Nkandla, most of whom lived in mud huts in extreme poverty.

We drove up the long steep pathway towards the hospital where there stood three armed guards. They quickly took a stance, pointed their guns at the car and started shouting angrily.

It was rare to see a car on the roads at this time of night, and David said they probably thought we were an armed gang of thieves trying to rob the hospital of drugs.

I looked at David for his lead, but the guards were beginning to shout louder and becoming agitated that we were not responding to them.

David stared at me in panic "Get out of the car." I looked at him, shocked, as he shouted again "Get out quickly, show them you are white." I understood, and slowly got out of the car with my hands up. I was probably the only white man for hundreds of miles, and a rare sight indeed at this time of night.

The guards approached me, shouting and waving their guns towards my face. Having survived this far, would I now be shot as a thief by a security guard? I knew they were telling me to do something but I couldn't comply with their request.

I could not speak Zulu and didn't have a clue what they were saying. I tried to stay relaxed, and smiled to display friendship, but it wasn't helping.

David quickly realised that there was a language barrier, and got out of the car to my aid. He explained I was from England and looking for a nun named Sister Hedwig. Thankfully, the guards knew her well and thought I was a doctor arriving at the hospital to work; and

I wasn't in a hurry to tell them otherwise!

They lowered their guns and raised the security barrier – and we drove into the relative safety of the hospital grounds with much relief.

Within a few minutes we found some English-speaking staff who explained they knew Sister Hedwig, but she was away and out of the area.

My heart dropped once more. Was my mission finally over?

David wanted to head back home fast, or at least find a police station to hole up for the night. But the hospital staff directed us to the convent where Sister Hedwig lived. Thankfully, it was next to the hospital.

David agreed to drop me there before he headed off, and we drove up to the convent, only to find it was locked down tight. Just like the hospital, it looked more like a prison camp than a convent in the dark night, with barbed wire and high security fencing. It took about twenty worrying minutes to gain someone's attention, that of an armed guard, who was patrolling the grounds and protecting the nuns and the convent from theft or worse.

The Sisters must have been fast asleep on my untimely arrival and were a little surprised to see me, given the remoteness of the area. One by one the Sisters woke, dressed and greeted me. They scurried around, somewhat disoriented, looking for their Sister Superior –

who alone would decide my fate – and if I would be given shelter for the night.

I introduced myself to nun after nun, and was greeted by the same look of surprise each time I did. I was desperately hoping they would not send me back into the darkness and dangers of the night, but by now the nuns had realised I was not Catholic.

As I met one of the older nuns, Sister Sola, I looked at her inquisitively for a second before involuntarily exclaiming "I know you," to my own shock.

"It is OK, God has sent you to us," she said, as if she recognised me too.

"I don't think so," I said under my breath, cringing with embarrassment at the thought. I felt really awkward now; I really did recognise her, although of course we could never have met.

Half of me wanted to leave the convent quickly, as it was no place for a person like me, but half of me wanted to stay in a safe place for the night and rest until morning.

As the Sister Superior approached I realised I had not washed or shaved for nearly two days, and was still wearing the same clothes I had left home in. The South African heat had not improved my appearance and, dehydrated and weary from travel, I must have looked and smelt awful.

Sister smiled at me warmly and offered me a room for the night, my taxi driver too if he wished. David was still sitting in the car outside and did not want to enter the hallowed grounds of the convent, or stay in Nkandla a minute longer for that matter. The nuns offered him some food and drink anyway and as a wide smile spread across his face, he quickly changed his mind and followed me inside.

Neither David nor I were churchgoers, but were trying hard to make polite conversation with the nuns who were in the process of setting out a banquet before us.

I had come to help a hungry child, not eat off the table of nuns, so took little food despite my hunger. David had no such inhibitions, and quickly piled his plate high with the plentiful meats and vegetables which had been laid out before us.

Suddenly I realised David was very uncomfortable. He was still and quiet and had stopped smiling. He was staring at his plate and I thought he was waiting for the nuns to pray, so I stopped too. Despite being hungry and thirsty, we both sat motionless in awkward silence.

A few seconds passed, and the nuns realised our discomfort and told us to eat. David, usually a cheerful and boisterous man, whispered softly "I don't know how to use a knife and fork." I looked at his massive plate of food, and then into his eyes. He stared back…but it was too late. We were both frantically trying not to laugh, but I was losing the battle. A broad smile swept across David's face and he burst out laughing. I tried to resist with all my might, but it was futile, and I burst out laughing hysterically, as tears rolled down our faces. One of the nuns stood up, desperately trying not to laugh herself, and smiled politely, before hurrying off for a spoon for David.

After this, the nuns accepted us for who we were with a gentle grace.

The atmosphere relaxed, and as we ate, I explained that I had seen the children's awful plight on TV a few days earlier and had felt compelled to travel here. We talked for a while and it wasn't long before I realised that this small convent of ten incredible nuns was the first, last, and only hope for the 140,000 forgotten Zulus who lived there.

The nuns estimated that one in four Zulus in the area were dying of AIDS, and said many were dying of TB too. Almost all the people lived in abject poverty in mud huts without water or electricity, and over 95% of the population was unemployed. Worse still, almost all the children were malnourished and many were orphaned due to the AIDS pandemic which had killed their parents.

Although Nkandla had one of the highest HIV infection rates in South Africa, there were no charities working here and the government was providing anti-AIDS drugs for just *ten* people. And these were only on a trial basis!

Why?

I didn't know, but felt despair at the inhumanity of the situation and the complete lack of response by the outside world.

The nuns did all they could to help people, comforting the dying and supporting the living, giving small food parcels to young hungry orphans whenever they could. But they knew they were losing the battle to save this doomed Zulu community.

I told them I had seen a young Zulu boy called Sne suffering on TV and had come to help him as I feared for his welfare. They said they knew of Sne's plight and had been trying to help him since his father's death, and if his plight had touched my heart in this way, much good would come from it.

For an instant the situation almost made sense.

After chatting for a while we were taken to a guest house which the nuns had prepared for us, and after my long tiring journey, to a destination unknown, I slept like a log.

I was awakened in the morning at 6 a.m. South African time (4 a.m. on my body clock) by the sound of angels singing.

It was the nuns, singing their morning hymns, a surreal moment for me at this unholy hour, yet despite my tiredness, strangely peaceful.

Where there's a will there's a way

Searching for Sne

I showered and dressed, and met an exhausted David, who had also been awakened by the singing and was now anxious to return home to his family.

He wanted to start the long journey back to Durban as the sun rose and offered to take me back, free of fare. I hadn't found Sne yet, but was momentarily tempted by his offer.

The nuns wanted to take me to the orphanage they ran to see some of the children they looked after. David knew he was my only way back out of Nkandla, and agreed to delay his journey home and come with me.

Despite being in the protection of the nuns, the intuitive sense of danger I had felt in Durban was ever present now. Indeed it was growing rapidly, and I found I was constantly telling myself I would not die here. Not this day.

We travelled with the nuns a short distance to an orphanage they ran and met 15 healthy, happy children; surprisingly full of life and energy, given their terrible circumstances. I was allowed to pass around tennis balls and other small toys; you would have thought it was Christmas, but then I guess it was to them. I played with the children for a little while with David, before the nuns lined them all up to sing traditional Zulu songs and dance, which they delighted in doing for us.

David was clapping, smiling and laughing and his infectious personality was encouraging the children to do the same.

It was 7 a.m. as we left, and the children were preparing to leave for school – I looked at David sadly, but we both knew these were the lucky ones. As we drove back to the convent we were told all the children had been given for breakfast was a cup of fruit juice. The carers had not woken up early enough to prepare breakfast for the children, and if we had not visited at that moment the nuns would not have known this was happening.

The children would not be fed at school and it would be evening before they would eat. Now the nuns knew of this situation they would take action.

I was furious with myself. Why had I not thought to bring bananas or food for the children?

The nuns took us back for breakfast; but knowing the orphans had only received juice for their breakfast and would receive no food until evening made me ashamed to eat – and I would not, despite the nuns' protests.

After breakfast the nuns offered to help me track down some of the families I had seen on television a week earlier. David was keen to set off, but again agreed to delay his journey.

After travelling into the hills we first found the Lindiwe family. It is hard to describe the contrast in the backdrop of the natural beauty of the area compared to the poverty and desperation of the people who live there.

Lindiwe was a destitute mother dying of AIDS, desperately trying to feed thirteen young children, many of whom she had taken in after their parents had died of AIDS.

We were invited into Lindiwe's traditional Zulu "hat" (hut) and she was lying on the floor, obviously very ill. The hut was small, containing only a bed, a small table and an old wooden bench.

Four young children were playing inside and as the nuns talked to Lindiwe I passed around some sweets, bananas and a few toys and clothes.

It was amazing to see the happiness this small act brought to their faces. The youngest child was nick-named Busy Bee as he never sat still, and we played for a short time, whilst David and the nuns chatted in Zulu with Lindiwe.

David was on his own mission by now. A mission to make everyone he met happy. To see him make Lindiwe laugh and smile was an enlightening experience for me, and one which made me realise what was really important in life – and what was not.

David interpreted for me (I hadn't even considered the language barriers when I had first left home). Lindiwe was becoming famous: as part of the TV documentary Sir Elton John had visited her and had sat where I was now. "Did he sing for you?" I asked. "No," she replied, smiling. Despite her awful circumstances she seemed glad her plight was bringing attention to the needs of her people.

As we were leaving I gave Lindiwe fifty Rand and she got up from the floor and started dancing around and smiling widely! The sisters told me that she sometimes had to save up for a month just to buy soap, and I felt ashamed for being able to do so little. Yet she was happy, and I had just witnessed the best cure you could ever provide to the sick – hope.

We rested for a while, sitting in the warmth of the midday sun, and I pondered how blind humanity had become to the plight of others around them. Where were the governments, the charities, the men of God and people of great power and wealth?

I knew children would die here today, out of sight, out of mind, alone and afraid. But who on earth cared…

The nuns suggested we try and find Sne. David agreed, and my negativity quickly changed to overwhelming excitement.

Although I had responded to the documentary immediately, it had been filmed over a period of many months and the nuns had been trying to help Sne and his sister Mbali since the death of their father. They told me they had at first placed the children with their uncle and his wife for safety. Sne's uncle, Simon, was a good man, but he had no income or employment and was impoverished. He lived in a mud hut without water or electricity, and often struggled to feed his own four children. Sometimes the family would have go to bed without eating that day, and taking in Sne and Mbali had strained the situation further, and things had not always worked out well.

Whilst it would be unthinkable in the western world, children in Zululand were often abandoned due to poverty if their parents died. Many orphans had simply become forgotten victims of a plague that was blighting the lives of millions of people, and they were left traumatised and victimised, without the love or protection of their parents.

I felt a sickening feeling grow within me as we continued to drive the dusty potholed roads, before finding a small school which Sne might be attending. As we entered we found each class was packed full with up to 140 children per classroom! The children stood toe to toe and could barely move; they had no desks or chairs, and little paper or pens to write with.

The sisters explained many had not been fed that day, and many were AIDS orphans who would have to beg for food to survive – or, worse still, do "child labour work", another term for prostitution. This would be horrifying in any community, but in the midst of an AIDS pandemic it was simply gut wrenching.

Yet incredibly, it would only cost a few pence to feed each of the children. I was struggling to accept the inhumanity of the situation, it was unforgivable and it had to stop.

I had only come to help one child. Now I realised Sne was one of thousands of children who desperately needed help.

Sne couldn't be found at the school and I started to worry for his safety again. As we continued travelling, I bought hundreds more bananas and gave them to the hungry children we passed on the roadside, and the nuns began calling me "Banana Man", along with David.

We kept travelling through the beautiful countryside passing rural homesteads with homes made of mud. Then, as if by magic, the Sisters spotted some children playing football in the open fields. Sne could be one of them.

The rickety car we were travelling in was not designed for off-road driving and I wondered how much longer the small car could navigate through the rugged plains. Nevertheless, we proceeded carefully in the direction of the children.

As we got closer, we stopped the car and the nuns got out and called to the children to see if Sne was amongst their group. At first there was little response, then slowly from the distance, a small figure started to approach us apprehensively.

It was Sne; I couldn't believe it! Having travelled thousands of miles to an unknown land, I had actually found the young boy whose plight had broken my heart just days ago! Finally, I was able to help him with food, sweets, clothes, toys and medicine.

Whilst I was with Sne, time stood still. The feelings of that moment are indescribable, save for the words of a great poet who captures them in a way I cannot:

To see a world in a grain of sand
And a heaven in a wild flower
Hold infinity in the palm of your hand
And eternity in an hour
- William Blake

We played football for a while and the nuns tried to explain to Sne that I had travelled a long way from another country to help him after seeing his plight on TV. Sne didn't understand, why should he? I was just some strange man who had appeared out of nowhere and had given him some food, clothes and toys. He was very happy for this and I knew he was safe now under the watchful eyes of the nuns. That was all that mattered.

Then, as quickly as I had met him, Sne slowly disappeared as he wandered off to play with his friends again.

We returned to the convent and the warmth and energy that flowed through me was endless. Knowing that Sne was safe, my mission was complete.

All too soon my journey was coming to an end. David, who had agreed to take me on a one-way journey into Nkandla (although he didn't know the way), had stayed with me now over two days, at no extra cost, acting as driver, interpreter, security guard, historian and father and friend to the hundreds of children we had met. But he wanted to return home to his own family now, and so did I.

If you can't feed a hundred children – feed just one
Mother Teresa

Back to 'Reality'

I wanted to return home, but I still had an overwhelming feeling that death was stalking me. I told 'death' that it had had enough blood in this land and to leave me alone – I would not die here; not today.

At the convent we said a fond farewell to the nuns, but as we were trying to leave they kept delaying us, to the increasing annoyance of David. They wanted photographs to show Sister Hedwig, the nun I had tried to find but not met on this journey. After various photographs they headed off to find some provisions for us to take on our long journey back to Durban. Then at the last minute they wanted to give me some traditional handmade Zulu gifts for my wife and children, and they promptly filled my empty suitcase with various items the local Zulu women had made.

Finally, we climbed into the car and the Sisters blessed us and said they would pray for our safe return home.

I promised I would send them a little money each month to help them in their work and to help them look after Sne. I would try to help them in any way I could back in the UK, but as the taxi pulled out of the convent, I had no idea how.

David was anxious to get going. The roads were still poor, but driving in daylight made us both feel a lot better. The roads in the mountains were treacherous, with sharp blind corners and deep potholes, which forced cars to veer to the other side of the road to avoid them.

We had hardly begun the journey homeward as we navigated such a road, and as we approached a corner, we saw that a car had recently swerved on to our side of the road and hit a truck head-on at speed. Two people had come through the car windscreen and lay dead on the roadside, others were lying injured. David looked at me knowingly, "If the nuns had not held us up for so long, it could have been us that the truck had hit," he said starkly. I looked at him and nodded, as a shiver ran down my back. His words provoked many feelings inside me. Had the nuns helped us cheat death; or was this just another coincidence in an ever-growing sequence of strange events?

I didn't know; but we were both very happy that the nuns had delayed us.

Help arrived, and we continued our journey. As we drove we passed many Zulus hitchhiking, desperately trying to obtain a lift along the roads. Despite the fact we had seen the crash earlier, there were few vehicles on the roads and most Zulus had no alternative but to travel by foot.

David would not stop for anyone, as he knew it was dangerous to let hitchhikers in his taxi. It was common for cars to be hijacked in this way in South Africa, and he knew many taxi drivers who had been robbed, shot or killed.

Just then we passed two young women carrying babies and I looked at David and shouted "Stop the car!" He looked at me pensively. I looked back and started to smile. "Don't worry," I said, "I'll protect you if these dangerous women with babies try to attack us."

David looked at me, smiling, then burst out laughing.

David dwarfed me in stature and was a large stocky man, powerfully built. Yet his socially embedded attitude had distilled fears in him that all hitchhikers were dangerous, and I think he had just realised that this was nonsense!

He stopped the taxi and reversed, beckoning the grateful young mothers to climb into his taxi for a lift, which they did readily. David spoke with them for a short time in Zulu and discovered that they were desperately trying to earn money to feed their babies and had heard of a place that might be offering work nearby.

It had been a misty morning and as we pulled away the heavens began to open and heavy rainfall fell. We drove for at least 20 kilometres before the women reached their destination, and I couldn't believe they were going to walk all that way, carrying babies in the torrential rain, just to find work which would pay a handful of Rand a day.

As they went to get out of the taxi they were so grateful they tried to give David the few pennies they had between them as a gesture of gratitude; he promptly refused and I got out of the taxi to help them out of the car, and gave them the last of my cash, so they could feed their children.

I got back into the car and David was smiling, "Look behind you." I turned inquisitively to find the women dancing in the road. David turned to me laughing "These women will be talking about you for years to come!" "What for?" I said, surprised by his comment. "It's probably the first time anyone has given them cash in their lives" he said. I felt myself shrink into my seat, feeling humble and small, as I had done so often on this trip of self-discovery.

I didn't talk much with David after that, and retreated to my thoughts, until out of the blue he said, "Kevin, God brought you to me." I looked at him in surprise, but knew how he felt. "No, I think it's the other way around, he brought you to me," I said.

Neither of us was the slightest bit religious, yet we both knew some strange force had brought us together. It was as if everything that had happened, had been in some way meant to be.

As weird as it sounded, when I looked back over time since watching the TV documentary, things had magically fallen into place one after another.

First, Joanne had set me free to come on this incredible journey. Then there were the strange coincidences that had happened to me when I went shopping in town. The three South Africans I had met in quick succession who had answered many of my unasked questions; the hundreds of pounds worth of clothes I had been able to purchase for next to nothing, and the small fortune in low denomination Rand notes I had acquired, being just what I needed in a third world economy. Then there were all the frustrating delays. Had these led me directly to David, who five minutes earlier or later would not have been standing at the taxi rank?

How the other taxi drivers had turned me away, leading me to him. If

I had been the proud owner of a credit card back in Durban, I would have hired a car, a fatal mistake which could so easily have led to my death.

Then I realised the importance of finding the nuns, as we had at night, and how they had taken me in at my time of need. I remembered the overwhelming feeling of familiarity when meeting Sister Sola. I still knew her now even as I reminisced!

Without meeting the Sisters I would never have met Lindiwe or completed my mission to find and help Sne, the very reason for my journey; and of course the delays the Sisters had caused us only a short time ago, which may well have saved us from a fatal crash.

I thought how travelling this very road, we had just met two women, so desperately needing a lift to find work to provide for their young babies. Was it all just one big coincidence?

I don't pretend to know, but it didn't feel like coincidence. Each event had led to another and been accompanied by a feeling of purity, and a deep emotional energy which made them feel so natural in occurrence, almost as if fated to happen, or driven by desire in some way.

The journey had changed David too. He said he would go back to Nkandla as soon as he could with sewing machines so the women could make clothes and earn a little money – this act of kindness was far greater than any I had made. I knew David was very poor himself and had a young family to feed. He would never own his own car; the battered wreck we drove was hired from the taxi firm, and he would never be able to own his own home either.

Finally, after many hours of driving, we arrived in Durban and I said good bye to David, a new friend, and a saint amongst men in my eyes. He desperately wanted to see his family again, and as I shook his hand with gratitude, he said he knew we would meet again in the future.

I knew he was right. One day we will.

Knowledge advances in steps, not leaps.

It doesn't make sense

My journey wasn't over, like David's was. He would soon see his family, but I had much more travel ahead of me before I would see mine. As I watched David drive away, my mind was still in Nkandla, and I vowed I would do all I could on my return home to help the forgotten children.

I entered Durban airport and walked into a different world: food, clothes, gifts – all for sale to anyone with money. I felt low, then intensely angry; why was the world ignoring the plight of the people only a few hours inland?

The happiness I had felt whilst in Nkandla was deserting me quickly and I was beginning to boil with grief and anger at the wealthy, neglectful scenes all around me.

I walked around in a daze for a while before inadvertently wandering into a private lounge, where I slumped into one of the plush seats. Anger was overwhelming me now, and adrenaline coursed through my veins as my mind raged to the point of exploding.

All I remember of this dark time is being approached by an aggressive businessman who had just been shouting abuse into his mobile phone. He had seen me in my dirty t-shirt and shorts and started to angrily tell me that I could not stay in the private lounge. I glared at him with contempt, my eyes welling with tears of torment. He stumbled backwards as he turned swiftly to walk away. They say the eyes are the gateway to the soul, and if he glimpsed into mine at that awful moment it must have been a terrifying sight for him.

This feeling of anguish was not passing and as I went to board my first plane home I stood on the tarmac looking up to the heavens, cursing that no God worked on this earth. As I stared skywards I saw within the massive plane engine above me a large Yin/Yang symbol. I had studied martial arts for over twenty years and knew that this symbol meant balance. Why it was there I do not know, but I immediately relaxed, my breathing slowed and I felt the overwhelming adrenaline pumping through my body dissipate, as I quickly calmed.

The rest of the journey home was very tiring – I had been on six planes in as many days – driven at least sixteen hours whilst I was on the ground, and not eaten or slept properly the whole time.

A day later I arrived back in Merseyside with the maddening knowledge that thousands of children were left orphaned, starving, frightened and alone - yet it would only cost pennies a day to help them.

By now I had no money left in the world, and the only asset I owned was my family home.

At home I greeted my relieved family. I had not been able to speak with them whilst in Zululand and Joanne had feared the worst. She burst out crying as she threw her arms around me.

Apart from the relief of me returning to her, I looked tired and ill and had lost over half a stone in weight in just a few days. I told her my many amazing stories and how I had found David, the nuns, Lindiwe and finally Sne.

As I spoke she knew I had changed; and she was right.

If I had left home under a cloud of madness, then I returned home *Bananas*.

Poverty is the worst form of violence
Mahatma Gandhi

Changing Times

I don't believe in Karma – but I was about to experience it anyway.

Ironically, having successfully avoided catching AIDS, TB, malaria and a host of other deadly diseases in Africa, I had caught food poisoning from a piece of chicken on the flight back to Paris.

I spent the next week in bed recovering, and despising travel anyway, promised myself I would never get on another plane again.

Slowly but surely I regained my strength. As I did, Zululand was constantly on my mind. I may have come home, but a part of me was still there. But by now life was forcing me to face my everyday problems again. We were having increasing problems within our road with the ever-growing presence of drug dealers, drunks and louts – and I wanted out fast.

But our savings were gone, and we were stone cold broke; yet deep inside I felt richer for my incredible experiences.

My small terraced house with large mortgage had been up for sale for over 12 months now, but not surprisingly, hadn't received much interest, given the problems in our road.

Our family home was our only asset now, and I knew if we could sell this it would improve our financial position and release some cash.

A few difficult weeks passed, leaving me feeling helpless to protect my family, or the children I had left to their fate in Nkandla – then, as if by magic, my luck began to change beyond my wildest dreams.

I bumped into a lady who had helped me a few years earlier when I had separated from Joanne after suffering a short breakdown in our marriage.

She was a landlady with numerous rental properties and had taken pity on me, providing me with a cheap roof over my head when we had separated.

She had become wealthy through property development and had just acquired her dream home – but then found it wasn't the right time for her to move in – so put it up for rent.

She was always on the lookout for small rental properties and I told her my house was for sale. She enquired where we wanted to live when we sold our house and I said we didn't really know yet.

We'd had so little interest from buyers that we had stopped planning our move, and house prices were rising so quickly it was becoming difficult for us to climb up the property ladder to a semi-detached home with a garden anyway.

After speaking briefly we chatted about life and Joanne told her about my antics in Africa a few weeks earlier. She was keen for someone she knew to look after her new home and asked us would we like to 'baby sit' it for six-months or so whilst we all considered our options.

Did we want to look after her house? Did we ever!

Two weeks later we moved from our small three-bedroomed terraced house to a half-million pound, five-bedroom, five-bathroom home, with about an acre of mature woodland gardens, private drive, courtyard and double garages!

As we drove up the driveway it was the first time my children had seen the house and they couldn't believe their eyes. As we walked through the doors we thought we had won the lottery. And so did everyone else we knew!

It was beyond our wildest dreams; beyond belief.

It was early April and the garden had just begun to blossom. My children, who hadn't been able to play in the street safely that morning, were now playing in secluded gardens, chasing squirrels, collecting pine cones, and exploring their new playground paradise.

James was in his element, and spent every waking hour exploring the gardens. Rebecca settled quickly too. If she wasn't in the garden, she was in her new bedroom with its 15 foot en-suite playroom.

Everyone was happy, and the peace and tranquillity was incredible. Wood pigeons, squirrels, hedgehogs, foxes and even two resident bats were now our neighbours – and the drunks, louts and drug dealers became a distant memory very quickly.

On top of this, just two days after we moved home, a children's charity acquiring investment properties in the area bought our now vacant terraced house.

A few short weeks later, the sale was completed, and we were mortgage-free and had money at our disposal for the first time ever!

Life was good. It was better than good, it was fantastic!

Joanne was quickly planning what we could do with the proceeds from the house sale: pay off some debts, a holiday to the Bahamas, a new car perhaps, new furniture and more.

Joanne's sister was getting married in the Bahamas in August and we had had no real chance of taking the two-week trip of a lifetime before our house had sold. Now she desperately wanted to see her sister wed, so we agreed to go.

But Zululand was never far from my thoughts and I knew I had to return.

Going Bananas

The children's plight had affected me deeply. Even after moving to our fabulous new home I would often break down in tears for no reason – unable to accept that an orphaned child was starving and I was helpless to prevent it.

Was I having a midlife crisis, becoming spiritually aware, or simply turning into a decent human being? I didn't know. And I had no one to turn to for help.

My family was not close; my own father had disowned me many years ago, a blessing in itself given his aggressive, unpredictable nature. And as for my friends, they would never have understood. I was heavily into martial arts and we enjoyed fighting and drinking; they would have laughed themselves stupid if they knew that ten Catholic nuns in Africa knew me as 'Banana Man'!

So I told few people, not even my family, and I began to feel very isolated. I knew children were dying, dying right now this day. If I went to Nkandla – if I was there this very moment, I could save them – but I was not. I was at home, or at work, and it seemed so very wrong.

I had not met Sister Hedwig on my first visit – the nun I had seen in the documentary – but she had been in contact with me by post since my return to England, and would occasionally email me from the hospital where she worked helping children.

We talked as if we had known each other a lifetime, and I quickly realised she used our conversations as a pressure valve to let off some steam and unburden herself from what she was living through daily.

email from Africa....

Dear Kevin...
.......It is hard, people are dying. I also lost a 2nd brother last year and the wife is sick and they have four children......It is not only my home, others suffer the same fate...

It was June now and the amazing coincidences that had happened to me through the year were occurring regularly now, but bizarrely they had taken the form of reoccurring numbers, which I would see everywhere.

If I dared look at a clock it would always be 11:11, or 1:11, 2:22, 3:33, 4:44 or 5:55. It was funny at first, but after a while it was happening day and night and beginning to drive me crazy. I would wake up at night from sleep and look at the clock and it would be 4:44am.

Why?

Whatever the reason, it was starting to annoy Joanne. But it wasn't just numbers. As I started to think about doing certain things, big signs would jump out in front of me as if the universe itself was saying YES do that. I felt like I was losing my mind and living in a pressure cooker that was about to explode.

Joanne was trying to look forward to going on holiday to see her sister get married. But I just wanted to get back on a plane and help the children in Zululand.

I had started going to the gym regularly to get in shape for the holiday, and the gym had TVs showing various programmes whilst you train.

Bizarre signs seemed to have been guiding me back to Africa for weeks, but today they were stronger than ever.

As I ran on the treadmill my mind wandered and I began to think about Zululand and the school I had visited, and the dying children there. As I did I glanced up and saw the news headlines on the TV in front me.

A news alert came on; school children in Durban had been attacked in the ocean by a shark. At least one child had died, and the clip showed a map of South Africa, circling Durban.

A shiver ran through me. I had just been thinking of school children dying in South Africa moments ago. I felt shocked, and got off the treadmill for a drink of water to cool down and collect my thoughts.

The news clip brought back vivid memories of my trip. How I had gone to help Sne and met Lindiwe. I hadn't heard from Sister Hedwig for a while, but last time we had spoken by email, Lindiwe's condition had been deteriorating.

I returned to the treadmill and glanced at the news again, only to see Sir Elton John giving a press interview! He had visited Lindiwe's hut as had I, and it was as if my desire to return to Zululand were receiving subliminal prompts from an invisible force telling me to return!

The news had spooked me quite badly, so I decided to go home; I showered and dressed and left the gym in a bit of a daze and got in my car. I started the engine and looked at the time; it was 11:11 am and I laughed crazily, as I was seeing this kind of number everywhere I looked.

I pulled out of the car park but my mind wasn't on the road and hadn't seen the other car in front of me and had to slam on the brakes heavily to avoid hitting it. It carried on before stopping at the lights ahead and I gingerly pulled out and came up behind it slowly. As I did I noticed its registration number; the last three letters said SNE - and I knew I was losing my mind to madness.

As I drove home my body was on fire as if my inner energy was bursting out of it in all directions. I knew I had to return to Zululand…and I had to return now.

I returned home and confronted Joanne in the kitchen. "Joanne, I have to go back to Africa," I blurted out, barely able to speak. "I don't know why, I just know I have to go back."

I started to tell her what had happened to me in the gym, and as I did so an Elton John song came on the radio which was playing in the kitchen. I looked at her with my hands wide apart, questioning my own sanity at the signs which were all around me.

She looked at me knowingly then said, "Go back to Africa and get this out of your system, then return home to me."

A few days later, I was standing in Nkandla once more, feeding children and starting another incredible journey...

Return to Africa

I hated long-distance travel, I really did. Having vowed never to fly again after my painful experience in February, I was about to endure the same journey again after only twelve weeks.

Those twelve weeks seemed like a lifetime to me. So much had happened and I was a completely different person, something my family was finding difficult to cope with. I had been on a mission to save just one child on my last journey. This time I intended to help many more and was able to take more money after the sale of our home.

If my first journey had been one of self-discovery, then it had been taken in blissful ignorance of what I was embarking on. Unfortunately I had no such luxury this time; I knew exactly where I was heading and how dangerous it would be.

As I arrived at Manchester Airport to check in, thoughts of worry started to race through my mind. Would I ever see my family again? I pictured James' face. He had been sad and tearful as I had left him. Joanne had been crying too and had not been very talkative, and Rebecca, as ever, had put on a brave face, although I knew she would miss me the most.

I remembered too the feeling that death had been stalking me on my last trip. Was I crazy? Why was I doing this again? Why did I not just send the nuns some extra money and get on with my life? Deep inside myself I knew why I was going back – but could I really beat the odds and make this perilous journey again successfully?

I spent the next two hours in the toilets being sick at the thought of what was awaiting me and dreading the travel.

When I eventually boarded the plane I settled down. I was flying from Manchester to London this time, then on to Johannesburg, before finally getting to Durban. The engines soon roared into life, and the plane took flight.

The day had been dull and overcast, but as we broke through the grey clouds the sunlight burst through the cabin window and blinded me with its brilliance. I pondered this event for a moment, realising that the sun was always shining, even when you can't see it for the clouds. This made me smile for a moment before I relaxed with feelings of serenity.

I'd never flown into London before, but it wasn't long before I departed the plane and prepared for my connecting flight. My mind was starting to adjust to my mission, and I felt out of place in the wealth and opulence of the expensive airport surroundings. I watched people milling about, some preparing for a summer holiday, others for business trips – and for a second I wished I was in their shoes; because I was preparing myself for a trip back into hell.

I bought a cup of coffee and found a seat. I blew on the coffee gently, then stared into it with a great sadness, knowing it had cost the same amount of money as it would to feed fifty malnourished children in Zululand.

I'd been dreading the overnight flight to Johannesburg from the moment I booked my ticket and had already accepted that I would not sleep again until I reached the convent in a day and a half's time. As the call was made to board the plane to Johannesburg, I contemplated my actions, shaking my head in disbelief that I had embarked on this crazy journey once more. I made my way to my uncomfortable economy class seat, and tried to settle in for the long haul ahead.

Despite my reservations, the flight was going well. I had watched a couple of movies and time seemed to pass quickly, and unknown to me I was also about to have an incredible night's sleep too.

What I dreamt during the flight I don't know. But it was the kind of dream I had rarely experienced before. It was a deeply pleasant, happy dream and one so funny that it was making me laugh as I slept. In fact I laughed so hard that it eventually woke me from my slumber. The lady sitting opposite had been watching me in amusement and was giggling so much herself, that others had noticed me laughing in my own private dream-world. As I woke, she looked to me, smiling, "You were really enjoying that" she said. Still a little disorientated, I looked at her a little embarrassed and said "Yes".

I felt mentally refreshed, and it seemed my soul was happy, even if my body was not coping well with the flight.

Time had passed quickly, I had slept soundly through most of the night and it was soon morning. Before long we descended towards Johannesburg, and I witnessed the contrasting scene of wealth next to poverty again. It wasn't a case of *déjà vu*, having first witnessed this bizarre paradox just weeks earlier – it was a stark new sight, and one linked with personal new experiences of knowing what it was like to be living in both of these camps.

I collected my luggage and a bag carrier offered to take my suitcase to the departure terminal for my final flight. South Africa portrays itself outwardly as a first world destination of tourist delights – yet as we walked, my slender built bag carrier begged me to give him my trainers. I felt awkward and tried to explain I needed them myself. He asked when I was leaving South Africa, and could he have them when I journeyed home. I politely said no and gave him fifty Rand for his help, and he left smiling happily with his tip.

I soon boarded my final flight, knowing the long drive through Natal would be much easier this time in daylight.

The nuns had sent me an email saying they would try and send a driver to pick me up from the airport. I had made all my connecting flights on time, and knew there was a good prospect I would not have to taxi my way into Nkandla again!

The comparatively short flight was soon over and I departed the plane feeling the warming African sun on my skin once more. I was physically sore from the journey, but my spirit was alive with energy and I felt at peace with myself and ready for anything.

I collected my luggage and wandered out of the airport looking to see if the Sisters had been able to arrange a lift for me. No one was there, so I decided to wait for a little while whilst I decided how best to proceed.

After a time I saw a nun in a white habit and wondered if it was my lift. I didn't recognise her at first, but as she got closer I realised it was Sister Hedwig! We had spoken often by email, but this was the first time I had seen her in the flesh. I looked at her questioningly as she approached and was greeted with a wide smile of acknowledgement. "Kevin," she exclaimed, "it is so good to meet you!" As she spoke her voice was familiar and full of joy.

Despite the circumstances she endured, Sister Hedwig had an internal happiness that glowed from within her. As we drove we talked and talked and she laughed in delight each time she spoke.

We had been driving and chatting for many hours when we saw a fruit market on the roadside. I knew we would meet lots of hungry children as we drove the final leg of our journey into Nkandla so I asked Sister Hedwig to pull over.

The traders, desperate for business, each heckled me frantically to buy fruit and vegetables from them, placing fruit in my hands and struggling to secure my trade.

I bought from as many traders as I could, and the car was soon full of the smell of bananas, oranges, apples and pineapples.

Before long we set off again, driving slowly now, in order to pass out our bounty of fruit to the children we met.

By now we were about an hour away from Nkandla, and despite having more bananas than I could count, it wasn't long before the car was nearly empty.

Each time I fed a young orphan I was paid back in kind with a huge smile of happiness, and a humbling sensation that the trip had been worth the journey, even if I did no more than feed the hungry child I had just met.

I remembered the feeling of incredible sadness I had felt back at home, knowing children were hungry whilst I was getting on with ordinary life – and knew how feeding these kids for just a day, made a world of difference to them in the waking moment.

Sister Hedwig must have seen the glow of wonder on my face and turned to me   knowingly. "A child's smile is eternal," she said; she was right – despite their awful plight these children had found happiness and hope for one short moment, and to witness this is to see the world.

As we reached Nkandla town, we saw a group of men trying to hitch a lift, to look for work. I asked Sister Hedwig to pull over so we could feed them. She turned to me a little surprised. "These are not children, they are men." I looked at her and smiled. "These are big children and they look hungry – let's feed them." She laughed back "Yes, big children get hungry too."

We left the young men in their thankless search for work, knowing that at least today, they wouldn't go hungry. Sister Hedwig turned to me once more. "When you feed a hungry person, you fill their stomach with food, but their heart with hope," she said, her eyes wide and full of wisdom – and I knew she must have experienced hunger all too often herself as a Zulu child.

We were close to Nkandla now and I could feel it approaching the way you can feel the powerful roar of a river as you get closer towards it. We finally reached the convent and I was greeted by the warmth of the nuns who had been waiting patiently in anticipation of our arrival.

And I instantly felt at home.

Probably the Best Convent in the World!

I entered the convent to discover it was one of the Sisters' birthday, Sister Ellen, a qualified doctor who worked in Nkandla Hospital, looking after the sick and caring for children. The Sisters were having a small party for her and had set out some food and drink to celebrate. Sister Hedwig headed straight for the kitchen to eat, and I sat down to speak with the other nuns.

I was dehydrated after the long journey and the nuns quickly offered me a drink. There was a large jug of orange juice on the table and I nodded yes as they poured me a large glass.

I had noticed the table as I had walked in the room, which had been full of cans of some sort. I was the only one drinking the juice except Hedwig – and the other nuns were sipping from the cans, but I couldn't quite work out what it was.

We were deep in conversation by now and I was the centre of attention, having just arrived, but as I sipped my juice I was beginning to look at the nuns in growing disbelief.

The small cans had writing on them – and I was trying to convince myself of what I was seeing.

It was Saturday evening. On a typical Saturday I might be out drinking with my friends, yet here I was, sitting in a convent in

Zululand, drinking orange juice, whilst the elderly nuns around me were drinking cans of beer and glasses of wine!

I started laughing, to myself at first, then openly to the nuns. I looked at Sister Michaelis and Sister Sola, who were sitting next to me, and they must have read my thoughts. "You like beer, Kevin?" Still laughing I said "Sometimes, and you?" "Oh yes, we are originally from the Benedictine order in Germany, who are master brewers. It is part of our diet here and good for your health."

"Wow, this is probably the best convent in the world," I joked to myself, as Sister Michaelis quickly replaced my watery juice with a cold can of beer!

The party continued for a number of hours, and as their guest, the nuns ensured my glass never ran dry. They of course never got drunk, and would drink maybe one or two cans of beer tops, but I was well into my fifth can and second or third glass of red wine, when a bottle of Amarula appeared on the table, for a nightcap.

The nuns were telling incredible stories of their youth, and as I looked at their elderly faces, they transported me back in time to their childhood – some had lived through the hardship of poverty and of the world wars – yet they told their stories with humour and grace. Many had been impoverished themselves in childhood, and some had been working at the convent in Nkandla since the 1930s – forty years before I had been born! As they reminisced I saw them as children with hearts full of joy, and realised we were all still children at heart, lost in the world and searching for meaning.

It was a unique experience to sit around, having a laugh and drinking beer with the nuns, but a rewarding one. And despite the fact I was not of their faith, they accepted me fully for who I was, and I felt at ease with them.

Slowly but surely I was beginning to wilt, partly from my long journey, partly from the drink. It was getting late, so I carefully rose to my feet, wished the nuns a good night, and walked slowly from the room.

Outside I stumbled drunkenly across the courtyard in the darkness, trying to find my way back to the guest house, muttering a feeble apology to God for being drunk in his house.

I found the guest house and unlocked the door after a few failed attempts. It was dark inside and I struggled to find the light. I then walked into a solid wooden table. "Ouch," I cried, more in annoyance than pain, before finding the switch and flicking on the dim light.

My case had been brought into the guest house by the nuns and I slung it aside and made my way to bed.

The African sun had long been replaced by a bright moon and the evening was cold. I shivered and climbed into bed fully clothed to stay warm, but noticed to my shock I wasn't alone.

The room was already occupied. Occupied by unpleasantly large local insects, which were crawling all over the walls and ceiling. For a minute I thought of jumping out of bed and squashing each of them to a pulp.

Then I realised, this was their home, not mine. I was the stranger here, not them.

So, as only a drunk could, I wished them all good night, turned over, and fell fast asleep.

More than enough is too much

Mission of Mercy

I woke in the morning with a slight headache and remembered quickly why I had returned to Nkandla. I had come here to work.

I walked into the main convent and met the nuns. "Would you like some breakfast?" Sister Hedwig asked. I didn't - but nodded yes out of courtesy anyway. The nuns were talking among themselves now, making plans for the day ahead. I sat contemplating how many hungry children were in the surrounding area, and felt sick at the thought; so ate only a small dry piece of bread in angry protest to the ridiculous situation around me.

The sisters wanted to take me out into the valleys to meet more children and I was keen to set off and find youngsters and help them.

We headed to the local market first, so I could buy some supplies of fruit to pass out as we travelled. By now it was a standing joke amongst the nuns to call me 'Banana Man' – which they did lightheartedly.

Sister Hedwig would be my personal chauffeur for the day and I met this news with excitement and fear. I was excited that I could spend the day talking with her and tracking down needy orphans. But Sister Hedwig's driving skills were erratic, if not dangerous – I had lost count of the number of locals she had narrowly missed on the drive into Nkandla. She would often drive at people walking the narrow roads and tracks, beeping her horn hysterically to make them move, which the majority did at frantic speed!

The roads here were for cars, not people – and it was their duty to move!

The main market was situated only a stone's throw from the convent, yet we had barely avoided hitting three people by the time we arrived there.

The stalls in Nkandla are manned by locals desperately trying to scratch a living. Sister Hedwig knew some of them well and guided me to the ones which needed the business most.

I duly obliged and it wasn't long before her small car was brimming with fruits, vegetables, eggs and bread.

Sister Hedwig was laughing and clapping as we practically bought the entire stock of one of the poverty-stricken traders, who seemed bemused but delighted by this rare experience.

We headed out of town and I watched the countryside roll past in awe.

As we drove we passed many hungry children and fed as many as we could whilst our supplies lasted. We had bought so much at market, yet the car was soon emptied, such was the need.

As we drove I looked out of the car window. It was the second time in twelve weeks I had witnessed the breathtaking beauty of the vast Zulu landscape, set against the backdrop of an unfolding human tragedy of a deadly pandemic, which was slowly eradicating the impoverished Zulu nation.

My mind wandered for a moment. In the news back home there were reports that a potential bird flu pandemic could sweep the globe, killing millions. I looked around me in anguish. If Zululand was an example of how the world responded to a pandemic, we were all in real trouble!

Over two million children orphaned in South Africa alone by AIDS. The government was in denial of the problem and the rest of the world did little, but ignore the plight of the ordinary people. Twenty million people had died worldwide since the outbreak of AIDS in the eighties. This despite the fact that drugs existed to indefinitely extend the lifespan of an infected person. Money seemed more important than life to the people in power. What a crazy, messed-up world we had created…

"Kevin," Sister Hedwig said, breaking me from my thoughts. "Yes," I said, as I turned to her. "We are heading to see the Nbula family now; it's a family of four young orphaned girls - their mother died in their hut. They sat at their dead mother's side for three days, not knowing what to do – then walked a whole day without food or water to find me."

We were driving offroad now and Sister Hedwig's battered old car was taking a pounding on the rough terrain, as it did daily. As we bumped and jolted within the car, she smiled at me and said "When Elton John visited he promised me a new 4 x 4 to help me with my work." "That's brilliant!" I exclaimed.

"I may just buy one of his CD's again now," I said smiling. She smiled back but I don't think she knew what a CD was. In fact, I wasn't sure if she even knew that Sir Elton John was a famous singer, and I laughed to myself quietly.

As we reached our destination, we stopped short of the huts as the car could travel no further down the tracks. We got out and collected the food parcels the sisters had prepared, and some of the clothes and toys I had brought from England.

Heavily weighed down, we struggled the few minutes' walk and found the young girls at their hut. They were all ill with the flu and Sister Hedwig explained that flu was common here in the winter months because of poor diet. She looked at me standing in my shorts and T Shirt, red and burnt by the African sun, and with a broad grin on her face said, "Aren't you cold?" "No," I replied, laughing, "your winter is warmer than our summer." She shivered jokingly in amusement, then spoke with the girls as we passed out the food, clothes and toys.

I could only feel humbled as I looked at the delighted girls' faces. We talked a little and the Sister made sure they were OK before we said good bye.

As we drove away, I looked back at the eldest girl, now only seventeen herself, and my heart dropped in anguish; her appalling story was commonplace here, and I wondered how long before she became pregnant and infected by AIDS, and why on earth we allowed this situation to continue.

We had only been driving for a few seconds, when two boys waved us down from the roadside. Hedwig stopped and spoke to them in Zulu before bidding them to jump into the back of the car. It was Sunday afternoon – and they had just embarked on a long journey into Nkandla town for school on Monday morning!

It was about half a day's walk away!

They were both about fifteen, and orphans too. They lived at home only on weekends, and had to live with relatives during the week to attend the school, and would walk for hours each Friday to return home, and again Sunday to return to school for Monday morning.

"Kevin, would you like to see the Lindiwe family again?" asked Hedwig as we drove. "Yes, very much so," I said in a subdued tone. Sister Hedwig caught my mood and turned to me and said despairingly, "I wish I didn't have to see all the horrors here when I can do nothing to help, it would be best if I never saw them at all." I knew exactly what she meant. I felt helpless to do anything. Yet even the smallest of our actions - a loving smile, a kind word, a lift in a car - seemed to make such a big difference here. They gave something money alone could not provide to these desperate people: hope.

"There is no magic wand here, Kevin." I had sunglasses on but turned away from Hedwig, fighting back my emotions. "I will be a magic wand," I muttered to myself in anger. "I will be a wand".

I didn't want to talk anymore. I had brought my walkman and put on some loud club music to drown out my thoughts and hide inside myself. It's quite bizarre trying to block out the world around you in this way. As a powerful song by the group Sash, 'Stay', ripped through my ears, it only acted to burn intense memories into my mind. Memories the song still triggers to this day.

There I was, in the middle of Zululand, an area of incredible natural beauty, yet a living hell of death and disease, poverty and social meltdown. Driving with a Catholic nun and two impoverished orphans at breakneck speeds, dodging pot holes and people alike, passing malnourished children at every turn, and ignoring many people at the roadside begging for assistance. All whilst listening to Sash at deafening volumes. Surreal.

As we headed towards Lindiwe's homestead, we travelled down a hillside towards a very narrow bridge, crossing a small river. Across the bridge a young boy stood patiently waiting for passers-by, in the hope they would stop and buy some of the honey he was selling.

I pointed him out as we came down the hill and Sister said, "He's probably been standing there all day, but few people pass down this road in cars, and he will never sell honey in this heat."

I watched his face as we drove past him as if in slow motion, then shouted spontaneously, "Stop the car." Sister looked at me puzzled, then pulled over.

"He'll sell his honey today," I thought as I got out of the car and marched towards the boy. He was a filthy mess, even by the standards of others in the area. Hedwig was out of the car by now, following me. She explained that he looked such a mess because he had been crawling around the nearby farms, stealing the honey from the white landowners. Hedwig seemed angered by his 'sin', but looked at me and said "The farmers will shoot the children dead if they see them." "What about the police?" I asked. She shrugged her shoulders in resignation. "The farmers never get charged; they say they thought it was a wild monkey and pay the police a few Rand for their trouble."

"WHAT - that's a national disgrace!" I ranted, enraged.

It was obvious the boy had no other choice in life than to steal to survive. He was skinny and gaunt and he had to steal food to eat. He was an orphan and probably had young brothers and sisters to feed too. I looked at Sister Hedwig. "Is it a crime to steal food to live?" "Yes, it is," she said pointedly. "Well, I'd steal to feed my hungry children if I had to," I said harshly. She looked at me briefly with disappointed eyes. "I would," I repeated without thought of guilt.

In her mind, she had thought me a righteous man, but this seemed to take her back a little. I didn't want to upset her religious beliefs, and knew one of the Ten Commandments she lived by was "Thou shall not steal."

I turned to her again and said, "Food is free. Does it not come from nature, and grow by the dynamics of nature through earth, sun and rain? Man may have put a price on food, but do you not believe food comes from God, not man? You can't steal from a man what is not his."

She looked at me questioningly, but didn't reply and I knew I wasn't going to change her mind, whatever I said.

We had reached the young boy by now and I saw his day's 'steal'. I hated honey, I really did. And the boy had massive sticky pieces of it which he was desperately trying to put in my hands. "Thank you," I said, trying to pass it quickly to Hedwig who obviously wasn't keen on honey either. I only wanted a small piece as a token gesture to justify giving the boy some cash. I took a small chunk from him, and Hedwig laughed, "He wants to sell you the lot!"

The two hungry passengers we had picked up earlier had joined us, and I nodded to them to help themselves. They quickly grabbed large pieces of the honey and ate it, smiling and chatting in native Zulu.

Hedwig didn't want any honey, despite my attempts to offload the sticky piece I held, and I told her to tell the young Zulu boy he could keep the rest and sell it later. I reached in my pocket and pulled out a hundred Rand note and passed it to the boy as payment. He looked at it in utter horror and froze for a second. I was confused, but Sister looked at him smiling and said "It's OK" before turning back to me. "Kevin, this boy has no money in the world, he cannot change that amount of money, have you not a few Rand to give him?"

I looked at her in surprise, "I don't want any change" I exclaimed, "that's for him to keep for the honey." She burst out laughing and explained to the boy that the king's ransom he was gripping so tightly was his to keep. Still shocked, he turned and pelted away from us as fast as his young legs could carry him.

"He thinks you might change your mind, perhaps," said Hedwig, laughing uncontrollably as the boy disappeared quickly from sight.

It was a funny sight for sure, but I felt so small and humbled by this ordeal that I wanted to disappear into thin air myself.

We returned to the car and started to drive away. As we did our passengers were laughing and pointing out of the back of the car, so I turned to see what was happening. The young boy had returned to the roadside and was frantically eating the honey we had left behind.

He had stood at the roadside all day in great hunger, drooling at the sight of the sweet honey that he had risked his life to steal; now finally, it was his to eat!

"He is a very happy young man now, I think," Hedwig said.

She was right; and as we continued towards Lindiwe's homestead, part of me felt great happiness at having helped this young child – but part of me despaired at his circumstances.

It takes courage to grow up and become
who you really are
E.G. Cummings

Lindiwe Must Live

Lindiwe's plight had been worrying me greatly since I had first met her earlier in the year. I knew she was dying of AIDS and if she did, thirteen more children would be orphaned instantly.

I turned to Sister and asked inquisitively "How much is a course of anti-retro viral drugs?" She thought for a second then said, "Anywhere between £80 and £90 a month, I think. Why?" "Mrs. Lindiwe is looking after many children, and if she dies they will all be left to a terrible fate like the other orphans we've seen, I can't let that happen," I replied, "not at any cost."

We arrived close to Lindiwe's beautiful but impoverished homestead, and Hedwig said "Speak to Sister Ellen later, she is a doctor and knows more of these matters than I." "OK" I replied, and we got out of the car to start the steep trek downhill to the huts.

Despite the intense poverty here, Lindiwe and her children would always greet a guest with a smile. She quickly recognised me as 'Banana Man' and remembered the day that I had met her with David.

Sister Hedwig spent time chatting away with her in Zulu, establishing her health and that of her extended family, and I used the time to play ball with the children, who giggled with delight at the attention.

After some time we said our goodbyes – and the children ran up the hill to wave us off energetically. We had left the family food parcels, clothes and toys, but as we drove away I knew Lindiwe must live. We decided to returned to the convent and drop our passengers into town, and I was keen to speak with Sister Ellen now about Lindiwe.

It was early evening by the time we arrived and the Sisters were preparing for dinner. Sister Hedwig was busy telling the others about the boy selling honey at the roadside, and I realised how unusual it was for people to receive help here.

Sister Ellen was in the dining room and I sat next to her to talk. She was a qualified doctor as well as a nun and I wanted to find out more about AIDS. She took a very practical approach to sex and the spread of AIDS within Nkandla. I guess she and the other nuns had no choice. Despite the Catholic Church's view of contraception and sex outside of marriage, the Sisters would encourage the sexually active to use condoms if possible, as this reduces the risk of spreading the AIDS virus, thus death.

One of the Ten Commandments is 'Thou shall not kill' and AIDS killed; so they tried to stop the disease from killing.

Ummm, makes sense to me, I thought, even the Bible has opt-out clauses in case of emergency.

I turned to Sister Ellen. "Can you put Lindiwe on anti-retroviral drugs if I pay for the treatment?" I asked expectantly.

"No, Kevin, it's not that simple. Lindiwe has TB too, and besides, people cannot start an anti-retroviral course if their white blood count is above 200, as Lindiwe's is. Her white blood cells would fight against the treatment, not with it, and this could make her condition worse, not better."

I didn't understand. I just knew Lindiwe must live.

"Is there nothing we can do to help her live then?" I asked.

"What happens is God's will," said Sister Ellen. "Lindiwe is a Catholic now and her soul will be received in Heaven when she passes away."

"What?" I said in shock as I took in what Sister Ellen had said.

"What happens here is God's will," said Sister Ellen again.

I looked around the room at the nuns, each of them an angel in my eyes, and my heart dropped. In that moment I realised that the primary mission of the nuns in Nkandla was to save souls, not lives.

They didn't want Lindiwe to die, not for a second. But in their eyes the afterlife was eternal; mortal life just temporary, so saving Lindiwe's soul, and that of all others, was of greatest importance to them.

They would do all they could to relieve suffering and pain of course, and had dedicated their whole lives to doing so in this blood-soaked land; but it was their conviction that what was happening here was God's will and he would judge us all at the end of days.

They had passed the responsibility to God. But I could not.

I could see no god wanting the suffering that was happening here, no matter how mysteriously he moved. I sat quietly for a moment, feeling isolated as a great burden befell me.

I felt overwhelmed by the situation and the enormity of the task to save these people, and left the room.

Prevention is better than cure

Enlightenment!

I returned to the guest house and sister Hedwig followed me. "What is wrong, Kevin?"

What could I say? That I didn't have the same beliefs as the sisters and cared more about life than religion and the afterlife?

I looked at Hedwig. "Nothing, Sister, I'm OK, I'm just not very hungry." I paused for a moment then said, "Is there nothing we can do to help Lindiwe? If she dies thirteen more children will suffer terribly."

She paused of a moment "I know some people take booster drugs", she said. "They are a high mix of vitamins which help boost the body's immune system." My mood changed a little. "Where can we get these - how much do they cost?"

"You can get them in town, I think. They cost about 100 Rand for a three-month supply," replied Hedwig. "That's £3 a month," I exclaimed. "Yes," she said sadly, "they are very expensive."

She had misunderstood me, and I had forgotten the value of money here for a moment. Three pounds was a lot of money when you had nothing, but in my world it wasn't much.

"You will take me to buy some tomorrow, Sister." "Yes," said Hedwig, smiling as she understood my intention. "Tomorrow then," she said as she left me.

I sat quietly at the small rickety table in my room and decided to collect my thoughts by writing them down. I had been drawn back to Zululand on a mission. But I had left home uncertain what that mission was, or what I could do to save the children. After all what could I do? I was just one man. I had decided to try and help Lindiwe, and protect her extended family, but was this possible in the face of a killer pandemic?

I started to collect my thoughts. OK, I'm known as 'Banana Man' here because I feed kids fruit. Why do I do this? I started writing.

"Because the kids are malnourished, orphaned and have no access to food!" How can I do this? *"Fruit is readily available, nutritious, and cheap to me and the local fruit growers and sellers benefit from me buying from them."*

So to feed a hungry child with fresh fruit cost less than 4p a day and the local traders benefit from the money spent at their stalls. But how do I feed lots of children? I suddenly remembered the schools. Of course, that was it!

There must have been three hundred children at the local school, and three hundred meals at 4p a day was….I looked at my calculator in amazement…£12.

It would take just £12 a day to feed three hundred children school meals of fresh fruit! "Wow, that's achievable," I thought.

I continued writing. *Five days a week at school, is £60 a week and say four weeks a month – that's £240 a month to feed 300 children; per head that's less than £1 a month to feed each child!*

It would take less than a pound a month to change a child's life by providing them with the security of regular food. Feeding them through school would encourage them to attend classes and help them gain a vital education too – all whilst boosting the local economy by buying the fruit from the local traders!

"Bingo!" I exclaimed, still not quite believing how little it would take to make such a big difference.

This was what I had been searching for. This was the reason I had been drawn back to Nkandla – to set up Fruit to Schools schemes to help the children.

I would talk to the nuns about this in the morning. They would administer the scheme for sure, and the school would distribute the fruit to the children, so there would be no overheads or administration costs. Magic!

I was getting hungry myself now; I hadn't eaten properly since leaving home, but I didn't want to go back into the dining room, having left under a cloud a little while ago.

I looked in my belongings to see if I had anything to eat and remembered the guilt I had felt when I had entered the convent a few days earlier. I didn't know the nuns partook in drinking then, and had smuggled a bottle of wine into the convent in my backpack, knowing that if there was a God up there watching me, I was in big, big trouble.

I felt better knowing it was OK to drink in the convent and after a short battle with the cork, managed to open the wine.

It was a clear night and I wandered out of the guest house with a chair and sat on the porch sipping my prize, gazing at the stars in awe. Wow! I had never seen the amazing star formations of the southern hemisphere before.

The sky seemed packed with masses of stars, clustered together in heavenly beauty. I sat mesmerised for a while, then started to ponder what on earth had brought the mighty Zulu nation to the brink of extinction.

The first time I had ever seen Zululand was as a young boy watching the classic film Zulu, staring Michael Caine. How could I have known then that twenty-five years later I would be helping the people who had never fully recovered from this long-forgotten war, and who were now trapped in abject poverty, battling against a new enemy - AIDS.

Was this really the long-term result of war? It seemed to be across Africa. I wondered if the children of Iraq and Afghanistan would still be paying the price of war for generations to come, long after the 'liberators' had returned home.

What a mess we have made of the world…

I finished my wine and went to bed.

Seek nothing, find nothing

Back to School

I woke abruptly at sunrise to the sound of loud screeching from the wild poultry that were housed next to the guest house. I arose wearily, with hunger pangs, cursing the fowl, and hoping I could eat them for lunch to quieten their squawks.

As I came around, excitement grew that I could put my proposals to the nuns on how to feed children with fruit through local schools.

I quickly dressed, before making my way across the courtyard and through the convent's corridors to the dining room for breakfast. Suddenly my mood changed and I became consumed with guilt again as I knew there were thousands of hungry children outside the security of the convent.

I entered the dining area and was warmly greeted by the nuns. "Sit down, Kevin, please have some breakfast." But I couldn't, my stomach was already full. Full of guilt and despair and anger once more. So I only took a cup of tea, and sat with the Sisters.

As I spoke I became excited again. "Sisters, I want to set up feeding programmes with you, through local schools, to feed children with fruit. Fruit here only costs pennies and we can buy it from the local traders. If we distribute it through schools we can feed hundreds of children every day very easily."

The nuns listened carefully as I spoke and they seemed very impressed by the simplicity of the scheme. "Also by giving the children the security of regular food through school we will encourage them to attend class each day, and this will help them gain an education and a chance of a better future."

"Yes," said sister Hedwig, "many children go hungry here and I know the schools will readily get involved and pass out the fruits in class."

"I will send you money for the project every month if you can administer the scheme and ensure the local traders we buy from deliver the fruit directly to the schools."

The nuns spoke between themselves for a minute, debating the idea, then Sister Carola spoke. "Yes, we have wanted to feed children here for a long time and not known how best to achieve this."

Sister Ellen turned to me, smiling widely, "You truly are Banana Man."

My nickname wasn't going to go away, and although still embarrassed by it, I said 'yes' with a slight smile.

Sister Hedwig piped up. "I know the perfect school to start with. The principal is very kind and does all he can to help the children. We will go there after breakfast, Kevin, and see him."

There was no time to waste. It was the last day of my short stay in Nkandla. Later I would have to leave and start the long trek back home. I finished my tea and hurried back to the guest house to pack my backpack, before returning to find Sister Hedwig.

She had finished her breakfast by the time I arrived and was waiting for me by her car, smiling. "Phalane school is not far away," she said, "but let's drop into town first to buy some provisions and see if we can get Lindiwe some booster vitamins."

I had nearly forgotten about Lindiwe in my excitement. "Yes, we must get booster vitamins," I said.

As we made the short trip I looked at Sister. "How is your family now?" I knew she was only in her mid-thirties like me, yet her mother and father were already dead, and two of her brothers had died of AIDS. She looked back sadly and said, "I have another two brothers dying of AIDS and I fear for them."

We entered town to the noises and smells of the market. Cattle and poultry could be bought here, as well as fresh fruits and vegetables. We soon found a small shop which sold the vitamin boosters, but it was shut for the morning. "Damn," I thought.

Sister Hedwig looked at me. "I can return here later and buy the vitamins for Lindiwe if you wish." "Yes," I said, reaching in my pocket for some money. I gave her enough for a six month supply for Lindiwe, and the same for supplies for her two brothers. Hedwig started to thank me but I stopped her. She had spent her whole life dedicated to helping others and yet she needed so much help herself.

Sister smiled and turned to walk to market. I followed her, thinking what a cruel world it was that left such an amazing woman to suffer in this way. "When I return to England, I will try and raise money to pay for anti-retroviral drugs for your brothers." Hedwig seemed a little surprised by this, but thanked me again.

Next we headed towards the hustle and bustle of the early morning market. As usual it was packed with traders desperately trying to scratch a living, yet it was full of life as people chatted, laughed and haggled. We bought as much fruit as we could carry in the car, knowing we would soon pass many hungry children as we travelled to the school.

The traders happily helped us fill the car, before we drove off to the sound of Hedwig beeping her horn, as locals jumped for cover!

The school was only about twenty minutes' drive from Nkandla town, but by the time we had reached it, we had dispersed the fruit to many grateful children with the usual familiarity, and I wished beyond hope we could have bought more.

You never forget the smiling face of a child you have helped in this way; but at night it is always the faces of the children you can't help that haunt you, and like a coward I would try not to look at children we could not stop to help.

As we drove Sister Hedwig turned to me excitedly and said "We had an email from Elton John's AIDS foundation recently. I have been invited to attend a fund-raising concert in the UK with Sne and Mbali in a month's time."

"Wow, that's amazing news," I said. "Have Sne and Mbali got passports or clothes to travel in?" "No," said Hedwig. I reached for my dwindling pile of Rand and gave it to Hedwig. "Take this, the children will need shoes and clean clothes." Sister laughed with delight. "The children are both safe at boarding school now, but I will arrange a big trip out of Nkandla, and take them shopping."

"I guess I'll see you in England soon, then… but I think you should leave your driving licence at home," I laughed, but Hedwig didn't get the joke.

We continued to travel and it wasn't long before we pulled into the arid grounds of Phalane Primary School. From the outside the school looked like a first-world school, built as numerous brick buildings, but this disguised a third-world environment on the inside.

The school was overcrowded and each classroom was practically bursting at the seams with children. We walked through the commotion of break time, where hundreds of children were playing, talking, laughing and shouting, and many of them pointed at me as we walked through the grounds. We soon entered one of the buildings and Sister Hedwig spoke with a teacher we met, who promptly directed us to the principal's office.

Hedwig was more excitable than usual as she turned to me. "The headmaster's name is Mr. Mbatha. He is a kind man and will be happy to run this scheme through the school."

We entered the building and Sister started chatting with one of the staff in Zulu. She turned to me sadly, "Mr. Mbatha has gone out for the day – we cannot see him before you have to leave, but we can see the deputy head in a moment."

We were ushered into a small office and asked to wait a moment. Sister had explained to the receptionist that I had travelled from the UK to help children and wanted to set up a feeding scheme at the school.

This seemed to cause a great commotion amongst the staff, and it wasn't long before the deputy head, a well-dressed Zulu lady who spoke impeccable English, came into the room with three other members of staff.

"Welcome, welcome," she said as she shook my hand in excitement, before introducing me to the other teachers. Each greeted me as if I were royalty and I felt a little underdressed for the occasion, wearing my three-day worn t-shirt and shorts.

Sister Hedwig reiterated the reason we had called at the school and the teachers' excitement grew and grew as she spoke. Hedwig looked at me, smiling "It is rare for people to come and help here, let alone feed an entire school!"

I was becoming a little uncomfortable with all the attention, but was quickly led by the hand from the room to go on a grand tour of my newly adopted school.

The school was incredibly overcrowded and had just 11 classrooms, in which to cram an endless sea of young faces.

"I'd thought the school would hold around three hundred children," I said. "No," replied one of the teachers, "we have room for six hundred, but are very overcrowded and have nearly nine hundred children here. One packed classroom contains 121 children alone."

"That's nearly three times more children than I had thought," I said, knowing that my calculations for paying for the fruit had just been completely blown out of the water.

We continued around the school and the deputy head told me that the school had only two toilets and no canteen. "Most of the children here live in poverty, and many are AIDS orphans," she said. "Hunger is a big problem here."

As we walked the teachers looked at me and asked "Aren't you cold?" They were all wearing trousers and coats, obviously feeling the frosty winter chill of the 28 degrees heat of the Zulu winter. Hedwig sniggered, pointing at my white legs protruding from my shorts, a rare sight in these parts for sure.

After our tour we returned to the office to talk. Hedwig was keen to get the project started and said "I will oversee all the administration and arrange the delivery of fruit, and you must distribute it to the children each day and sign off for each delivery." "Yes," said the deputy head, "that will be no problem at all. Mr. Mbatha will agree to this, certainly."

Everyone talked excitedly about the project, but my head was still spinning with the numbers. I hadn't banked on feeding nearly 900 children every day. Whilst the group chatted I took my calculator from my backpack and started to check the numbers.

One of the teachers confirmed there were 886 children in the school. 886 meals a day, five days a week, say four weeks in an average month, twelve months a year; my jaw dropped. That's over 212,000 school meals!

"Joanne's going to kill me," I said aloud by accident, to the bemusement of everyone in the room.

A Natural Step

With all the talk of food, Hedwig was getting hungry and wanted to head back to the convent for lunch. As we set off she sensed my unease. "This is your last day, Kevin, let me take you on a detour and show you something very special."

"OK," I said quietly, and didn't speak much after that. I was still contemplating the commitment I had just made to the school and the hungry children there. It was small in comparison to their need, and I wanted to do so much more – but I was beginning to worry that I had bitten off more than I could chew.

There was only so much I could do alone, and I was spending the sales proceeds of our house fast. What would Joanne say? She wasn't going to be happy; I'd already spent thousands of pounds on this trip, not to mention our life savings on the trip before.

We hadn't spoken for six days now, and she was probably sick with worry too. Before I had left she had told me that she thought she would never see me alive again, and this had played on my subconscious continually.

The trip had been worth every penny, I knew that. But I felt I was in danger of letting my own family down, trying to support so many children in this way.

No, I decided. We were living in a fantastic house back home, and were preparing to go on a holiday of a lifetime soon. We would be fine. Thinking of home made me miss my family again, and I wanted to return safely to them now, having completed so much in such a short period of time.

Sister Hedwig broke into my thoughts. "People back home will support you, Kevin, when they know what you have done here. Trust in God."

I smiled. "Maybe," I thought, wondering why all the charities were based in the large coastal city of Durban, when the greatest need was here.

We headed up a hill through a particularly impoverished area just outside Nkandla town. The roads were extremely poor and the car jolted from side to side as we drove and I had to put my hand on the roof of the car just to stop bumping my head as we bounced up and down, swerving across the road to avoid the large potholes.

We passed another school. "Are children fed there, sister?" I asked. "No, the Government runs few feeding programmes in Nkandla. There are many more schools like Phalane."

I had no idea where we were heading, but as we came to a peak on the hill I looked out of the car window in silent awe. Ahead, far in the distance, two giant forests seemed to meet before falling away into a valley below. It was a sight of indescribable beauty. I had never experienced nature like this before and for a second, I forgot about the poverty around me as nature filled my soul with an uplifting energy.

"Wow," I said as we stopped the car and got out to take in the view. "Yes," said Hedwig, who was staring ahead too. "Come, we are not there yet."

We returned to the car and continued up the hill until, out of the blue, a huge building appeared on the horizon. It looked out of place in the surrounding poverty of mud huts and shoeless children, and was set back behind a large gated fence of barbed wire and electrified fencing.

We pulled up to the gate and Sister beeped her horn, a rare treat given that no one was in danger on this occasion! We couldn't see the forests or valley now because of the hill ahead of us, and waited a while before two Zulu attendants appeared and open the gates.

Hedwig spoke in Zulu with the young ladies for a second, then they allowed us through the gates and locked them behind us. They hopped into the car, and we continued to drive off-road for a short time until we neared the crest of the hill.

The forest and valleys were still obscured from sight and the surrounding scenery was little more than grass, earth and gravel. We climbed out of the car and I wasn't quite sure why Sister had brought me to this place. As she chatted with the attendants she walked ahead, beckoning me to follow them.

As I came over the hill I stopped dead in my tracks. We had reached the valley, and its beauty took my breath away. Sister looked at me, smiling. "This is my favourite place to come to rest and be with

God," she said.

I stood staring at the surrounding landscape and its immensity dwarfed me. We walked down the hillside where six luxurious apartments were built in the middle of nowhere, in the style of fabulous Zulu style huts.

Decking had been built out from each of the apartments, overhanging the valley below to give the feeling you were walking on air. I walked across the deck of one of the apartments to the balcony and looked down hundreds of feet to the floor of the beautiful valley below.

Zebra and springbok were grazing beneath me and a small river swept through the valley, fed by an incredible waterfall which glistened brightly in the sun as it cascaded downward. Above, in the distance, the two great forests seemed to come together as one, at a point beyond the eye, and were shrouded in a hazy mist that you could almost feel. The valley was alive with the sounds of nature, which enveloped the entire area for miles around.

I looked at Hedwig, dumbstruck. "I have never seen anywhere like this before, Sister". She sighed as if to release the daily pressures of her world to the winds, and gazed ahead peacefully.

Hedwig lived in the middle of a hell, yet somehow, she had found a private Garden of Eden to unburden her soul.

The attendants were keen to give me a tour of the luxury Zulu apartments and I entered a world I had not seen since Durban.

Luxurious living space, a fridge and microwave oven, an en-suite bathroom with shower, and a large double bed covered in traditional animal skins.

A far cry from the poverty minutes away from me, and sealed off behind large electrified fencing which swept through the valley for mile after mile.

I looked at Hedwig questioningly, "Why is this place fenced off in this way?"

"For the tourists," she replied, grinning. I looked at her, confused. "No tourists are going to come out here, or find this place," I said.

"I know," said Hedwig. "It is a token built by the Government to say that there are tourist facilities within Nkandla town. Few people will ever use these apartments, but the Government can claim they have facilities here."

I walked back outside and sat on a chair on the decking. Sister joined me and we sat in tranquillity, soaking up the warmth of the sun and absorbing the energies flowing through the living valley, and surrounding forests.

"You are one of few people on earth today who will ever see this place, Kevin." I smiled. "What an incredible thought," I said, still gazing around me in awe of the natural beauty.

Sister was right, few people would ever see this valley, not even the local Zulus, yet it was a place you could spend your whole life and die happily in peace.

I wanted to take pictures but had run out of film. Hedwig looked at me, "What a shame you have no film left." "No," I replied philosophically, "perhaps it will be the reason I return here one day."

Whilst I sat there everything in the world seemed so clear, so simple.

The hungry needed food, the sick needed medicines, children needed their parents and orphans needed loving families to take care of them. How little it took to make a difference, yet how complicated we could make things when we had no real desire to help.

We enjoyed the next half hour in peaceful silence, except for the sounds of nature which filled the air with an invigorating energy. After feeling so alone the night before, I now felt at one with nature and all that surrounded me.

Man belongs to the Earth;
the Earth does not belong to man

Small Acts, Big Changes

We set off back to Nkandla town, passing many needy children as we drove, who would each smile and wave in response to seeing us.

What an incredible day, I thought: I had fed hundreds of children, set up food to school schemes which would provide hundreds of thousands of meals to hungry kids over the next twelve months, and managed to put three people on booster vitamin drugs to help keep them alive.

Lindiwe would be OK, Hedwig's brothers too. Sne and Mbali were safe in boarding school now, and I could very well see them in England soon.

Today I had walked through hell, and then into paradise, two very different places, just minutes apart. My journey was coming to an end now, but it had been as incredible as the first time I had travelled to this amazing land.

We drove back into the convent to meet the other Sisters, and it was nearly time for me to leave for home.

Sister Eobarda, the convent superior, wanted to accompany me on the long drive back to Durban, and I welcomed the company.

I went into the convent for a drink and a snack before I left and the sisters gave me locally produced gifts and baskets hand-woven by Zulu women. We chatted about Phalane and I knew the Sisters would ensure the children would be fed each day now, under their watchful supervision. Sister Hedwig had arranged to return to the school tomorrow to see the principal, and assured me she would kickstart the scheme by the end of the week. Then the Sisters said they would pray for me each day.

I smiled at this, a little embarrassed at the thought, but the nuns continued. They would pray for me that I would convert to Catholicism; it was their conviction that only Catholics could be received by God, and at the moment, I was doomed to damnation in hell as a non-believer! They did not want this to happen, and would pray for me each day that I would become a Catholic.

I looked at them a little shocked, then told them to pray for the children here instead. I knew they needed the prayers more than me. Besides, I had heard the nuns singing, and if I ever tried to sing in church, I would certainly be condemned to hell for the terrible noise I would make!

Despite my light-hearted words the sisters would pray for me anyway; and in a few months time I would need all the prayers I could get!

The sober mood of the moment soon passed, but I had no desire to become a Catholic, or join any other religious group for that matter. Yet something inside me was stirring; and I was beginning to see life in a new way....

Soon it was time to leave, and having condemned me moments earlier; the Sisters now each hugged me and gave me their blessings as they wished me a safe journey home.

Be the change you want to see in the world
Mahatma Gandhi

Freedom to Think

The journey back to Durban was a long one. It was a hot, sticky afternoon and our driver sped over the narrow roads with more confidence than I, that we would not meet oncoming vehicles on the sharp blind corners.

Sister Eobarda sat next to me and we chatted about her beliefs and those of the church. She was a good, kind person. She would help anyone in any way she could. Yet she had very fixed views that the Bible said if you didn't believe in a Catholic God, you were condemned to eternal damnation.

This seemed a huge burden to her as she wanted no soul to be sent to a fiery hell, and was the reason she had dedicated her life to convert others to find salvation.

As for me, I attended church for births, deaths and marriages only… but my journeys into Zululand were certainly beginning to make me ask questions of myself. Who was I? Where did I come from? Was there life after death or a God with a grand design? Why was I here and what was I supposed to be doing with my life?

I didn't have the answers; but I was no longer willing to spend the rest of my life working a mundane job, simply to reach retirement as an old man, before slowly fading out of existence as my body and mind deteriorated with age.

This was the start of a new enlightening and frightening philosophical journey inward, which some consider to be a midlife crisis.

I'm not sure this is true, and I didn't think I was having a midlife crisis; but if I was, I hope everyone's experiences were as amazing as mine.

Sister Eobarda didn't question life philosophically. She was driven by an unbreakable faith alone now, and to raise questions was to question God's word, something she could not and would not do. Nevertheless, she entertained my questions in good spirit and tolerated me in my quest to understand more about the world around me and her beliefs about what was going on and why.

As the hours passed, the scenery changed back to that of a first-world country and slowly but surely the roads turned from track to tarmac. As they did, traffic appeared once more. Signs of civilisation steadily appeared and by the time we had reached the beautiful South African coast, we had returned back into the hustle and bustle of my world.

I stared out of the window looking past the golden sands of the beach to the warm waters of the Indian Ocean. The ocean shone silver as the bright sun reflected off it, and I wondered how many tiny separate drops of water made up this mighty ocean.

As I did, I thought of each drop of water as a person. Each separated from each other, then united together again as a great ocean to become one. As I pondered this, I realised all people had the same roots. We were all branches of the same tree. We came from, and returned to, the same place. And just like the drops of water, we could combine with, or separate from, a mighty ocean of humanity. We were one as a race, even if most of us didn't act like it most of the time.

The young children in Zululand were no different from my own children. They were exactly the same. They needed their parents as much as my children needed me. They had the same daily needs, hopes and fears. Yet somehow, we had let the children of the world down. We had become separated from them, distant to them.

Sister Eobarda interrupted my thoughts. "Kevin, we are approaching the airport now." I looked at her philosophically as the car pulled to a stop. "You will see me again, Sister. I will help you as much as I can when I return home."

She looked at me and smiled, but said nothing.

The long drive had taken its toll on us all and we climbed out of the car slowly, stretching out our limbs in relief. After a minute or two of stretching it was time for Sister and her fatigued driver to depart. She hugged me warmly and blessed me, wishing me a safe journey home.

I responded in kind, knowing she faced a long and uncomfortable drive back to Nkandla herself. Then I watched sadly as she drove away, back to her world of poverty and injustice.

A great roar ripped through my ears as a plane soared into the sky above me. My journey homebound had just started and my stomach turned as I knew I faced three planes and another day's travel before I would sleep again.

Worlds Apart

I walked into the airport and felt overwhelmed by the wealth, as I had done on my previous trip. People were meandering about the airport, drifting into shops and restaurants, spending money as if it were nothing.

They seemed unaware of problems that did not directly affect them ....unconcerned that the price of a sandwich could feed a hundred malnourished children for the day.

My difficulty now would be readjusting back to my own life. It had taken me weeks last time, and almost driven me mad in the process.

I didn't want this to happen again. I knew I smelled after the gruelling drive from Nkandla in the South African heat. I had brought few personal clothes with me on the trip, and had, instead, crammed my case with as many children's clothes and other supplies as I was able to carry.

I couldn't get on a plane smelling like this, so decided to go and buy a new top to help me readjust back to normality more quickly. I walked into a sports shop and looked at the shirts and t-shirts. One I liked was 100 Rand; that's a three month supply of life-saving vitamin booster drugs, I thought, fighting feelings of anger. How could I accept this economy again whilst I knew millions of malnourished children lived in this country, yet 4p would feed them for a day?

The cheapest top I could find was a rusty red striped shirt with mismatched black collar. It cost £4 and must have looked awful with my black jogging bottoms and dirty trainers, but here, now – I just didn't care.

As I continued walking around the airport the smell from the food courts was beginning to overpower me. I had eaten little since leaving home and knew I had lost a lot of weight. Fighting the knowledge that children were hungry, I succumbed to my compulsions and entered a restaurant.

Families, couples and businessmen were sitting at various tables, eating, drinking, and talking. It was difficult to accept this scene as normal, given the last few days. A waitress greeted me and guided me to a table and I slumped wearily into the soft seat. "What would you like to drink, Sir?" she asked. "Just water please," I replied in a quiet voice. "I'll be back in a moment to take your order," she chirped cheerily as she went to fetch my water.

I don't pretend to know how soldiers feel when they return home from a battle zone after a tour of duty, but I can only imagine that at some level they feel the same way I did then. It was as if I was seeing the world around me as a movie, and it wasn't real. Everything felt wrong, trivial and false. I knew somewhere else a real world existed where people were dying. I should be there helping them, not shopping for new clothes or sitting in a restaurant ordering food whilst people chatted happily in ignorance of what was happening all around them.

"Your water, Sir. Have you decided what you would like to order yet?"

My smiling waitress suddenly reappeared and I must have looked at her blankly for a second or two. "Sir?"

"Sorry," I said, "I'm just a little disorientated from all the travel."

What else could I say?

I wanted to find a megaphone and announce to the entire world that children were dying whilst they milled about in their daily lives and that they needed to stop what they were doing and go and save these children right now!

"Oh…..er… just a burger please," I replied.

The words echoed in my ears. I hadn't even left South Africa yet, but was already failing the children by trying to let go of their plight and return to my own life.

I sat in silence until my burger came, then began to eat it as if it were normal to sit in a restaurant and eat. Tears tumbled down my cheeks as I ate and I felt numb. I felt like I was in a dream and had separated from my body to watch what was happening around me. Physically I was sitting, eating the burger and acting out a scene of normality, but part of me was there in the background watching, witnessing, as reality unfolded.

I finished my burger, feeling full and sick. Dark clouds continued forming in my mind, until then, like a bridge back to sanity I saw a flash of my family.

Joanne, Rebecca, James – all smiling at me in happiness.

I had a family to return to and I had not spoken with them for nearly a week now. Were they safe; had James had an accident, did they need me when I was not there to protect them - instead thousands of miles away in a foreign land? I began to panic in worry.

I had to speak with them and make sure they were OK. Joanne would be expecting a call today and must have been worried out of her mind by now. I had so much to tell her: the things I had done, the children I had helped, the places I had seen…and the food to school schemes I had set up.

God, she was going to kill me!

I left the restaurant in a hurry to find a phone. I bought a phone card and tried to dial home a few times without success, pressing the wrong numbers in my haste to make contact again.

The phone finally began to ring, and my heart was beating faster with each ring. "Hello" said a gentle voice. "Joanne, it's me, I'm OK…are the kids all right, are you OK?" "Kevin," I could hear her voice shake as she tried to stop herself from crying in relief…"Yes, we're all OK, we've just missed you so much, I didn't know…I didn't know if anything bad had…"

"No, I'm fine," I said in relief that everyone was OK. "I'm safe at the airport now – I'll be home tomorrow….I'll see you all very soon."

"How was the trip, did you do what you needed?"

"It was amazing, but I can't talk now, I haven't much phone credit. Tell the kids I love them and I will see you all tomorrow."

I had made contact, to Joanne's great relief, and thankfully everyone at home was safe and well. I put the phone down and thought with dread of the long distance I still had to travel.

I really did despise travelling…

They that travel far, have many encounters

Home with Heart

Three tedious flights and a taxi-drive later, I arrived back home completely exhausted.

Joanne opened the door and burst out crying as she saw me. We held each other for a moment then I entered the house and collapsed on the couch. I had lost nearly a stone in weight and Joanne looked at me in worry. "Going to Zululand is better than going on the Atkins Diet," I laughed tiredly.

She laughed through her tears before wiping them away.

The children were in school and I needed to go to bed to rest. Joanne brought me a drink and I recounted the stories of the people I had met and how I had set up the simple fruit schemes through a local school which would feed hundreds of children each day. She listened intensely, then helped me to my feet so that I could go and rest.

I woke hours later as my children returned from school; they burst into the bedroom and dived on top of me. James wanted to play, Rebecca wanted to talk, I just wanted more sleep. They dragged me out of bed anyway and I knew I would soon fall back into normal life whether I wanted to or not.

I was in contact with Sister Hedwig far more now, and received my first email within a week of returning home.

email from Africa.......

Dear Kevin...

...Yesterday the 13th June 2005, the 886 children started getting fruits. You must have seen the joy by the children...

The school was delighted by the start of the project, but the principal said he refused to believe it until he sees a truck in front of the school with the fruit...

...This has never been done by anyone before...you are the first one to do such a thing in our community...

Tears were welling in my eyes as I read Sister's email. My journey was still raw in my mind and I knew how much the food would benefit each and every one of the 886 children who were now receiving it; but I wasn't crying for them. I was crying for the thousands more whom I could not feed - and I didn't know how to help them.

Sister Hedwig's email reaffirmed that she was coming to London with Sne and Mbali, at the expense of Elton John, to attend a fundraising concert he was performing. The concert wasn't long away and I couldn't wait to see Hedwig and the children again.

I was worried for Sne though. It was a long, tiring journey to the UK and how would he cope with seeing London, which is so very different from his impoverished homeland. I had walked into his poverty-stricken land and then returned back to the wealth of the first world. But he was doing the opposite, and would walk out of a world of poverty, only to be thrust back into it ten days later.

Hedwig had told me that they were to be flown first class, which was fantastic news. But I couldn't help wondering how the money to fly them all the way to the UK first class could have been used better to improve their lives back in Nkandla instead.

It was late June and my family were enjoying the large gardens that our new home offered. Joanne wasn't over impressed that I was taking a two-day trip to London to see Sister Hedwig only weeks after I had returned from Africa – but we were going to the Bahamas soon for her sister's wedding and this pacified the situation.

Sister Hedwig had been invited to stay in London with the film producers of the documentary that I'd watched back in February, and I agreed to meet her there a few days after she had arrived.

The three-hour train journey to London from Liverpool seemed short in comparison to my previous travels. Life had been hectic since I had returned from Africa and it seemed like everyone had taken a piece of me until there was nothing left. Joanne, my children, work, friends, sports – they all needed my time and energy, and I felt burnt out.

I had wanted to put my energy into fundraising when I had returned home, but life kept distracting me from my task.

Today was different though. The journey to London was giving me time to relax and re-focus my thoughts. I was staying in London overnight and meeting everyone in the morning.

It wasn't long before I reached the hustle and bustle of London metropolis and found a cheap hotel room for the night.

In the morning, after a short tube ride and a brief walk, I found the film producer's house in the suburbs. As I approached I could hear Sne playing happily in the garden at the rear of the house and soon found Hedwig and the children. Everyone was enjoying the unusually hot summer's day, which rivalled the weather of South Africa in spring.

"Kevin!" exclaimed Hedwig, "It is so good to see you again. I am thousands of miles from home yet I'm meeting my old friend here." "Hey, less of the OLD," I said, laughing as we hugged.

"How are you, Kevin? Sit down with me. The Sisters send their blessing." Sister smiled with each word she spoke, a rare quality in people nowadays. "I'm fine, sister," I replied. "And you, and the children, how were the flights?"

"The flights were fine, we flew first class," she said proudly "and the children slept on the planes." "That's great," I said, relieved, "I thought you may have struggled with the travel."

I had brought gifts and sweets for Sne and Mbali and quickly passed them out to them.

Sne wanted to play football with me, and for the next half hour or so we played   together without a care in the world.

Hedwig and Mbali sat chatting and laughing as Sne ran rings around me in the summer heat, both refusing my attempts to have them join in to give me a much-needed break.

After a while I collapsed on the patio next to Hedwig, sweating profusely as she poured me a drink and I got my breath back. "How are the children in Phalane school?" I asked "Is the project going well?"

"Yes," said Hedwig, "it is an extraordinary thing you have done there."

"Extraordinary?" I laughed. "No. Isn't it ordinary to feed a starving child?" As I spoke I realised for some reason it wasn't ordinary anymore, something, somewhere had gone dreadfully wrong.

Global statistics showed that an incredible 800 million people did not have enough food to eat each day. Yet there was more than enough food in the world to feed us all!

"When it becomes ordinary again for mankind to feed starving children, what an amazing world we will live in," I said, smiling at Hedwig sadly.

Sister nodded. My words seemed to strike a chord with her too – we both knew the awful reality that we did leave helpless children to starve, to die.

We sat in contemplation for a moment, then I remembered I had brought Hedwig some gifts too. "Sister," I said excitedly," I have brought presents for you too."

She clapped her hands in delight. Coming to London was a trip of a lifetime for Hedwig, who had lived her whole life in a world of despair, yet for the next ten days I knew she would be able to relax and recuperate. She rarely received gifts of any kind and waited in excitement whilst I fumbled around inside my backpack.

I knew I may not see Hedwig again for some time and had brought her some money to help her over the weeks and months ahead. "Here's some cash to buy more booster drugs for Lindiwe and your brothers when you get back home."

"Spend the rest on Sne and Mbali and yourself whilst you're in London and take what is left home and use it for your work." Sister wasn't used to our expensive economy yet, but I knew she and the children would need some cash to enjoy the week ahead.

I reached back into my backpack and pulled out chocolates and a Life Diary and gave them to Hedwig. "A Life Diary lets you record your life story," I said. "You can record the key events of your life, and important stories you want to remember."

Hedwig looked at me in delight. "I have wanted to write down all my stories, so that I can tell people what I have lived through," she said. "This is perfect, thank you."

As she tucked into the chocolates, reluctant to share, we chatted more. The film producers joined us for a while, and we all reminisced about Nkandla with Hedwig and Mbali. Then I played with Sne again, until eventually it was time for them all to leave for Elton John's concert. And time for me to leave for home once more.

I said goodbye to Sne, not knowing when I would see him again, but Hedwig promised she would email me regularly from South Africa with updates.

As I sat on the train travelling home, I realised that if Sne and Mbali ever met me again in the future, they probably wouldn't even recognise me. I knew I was just some strange guy who occasionally turned up out of the blue to help them a little, before disappearing again just as quickly as I arrived.

As the train sped along the tracks, I watched the scenery roll past from the carriage window and thought how Sne and Mbali would never have the amazing opportunities available to me. As I contemplated this I realised that so few people around the world actually had the opportunity to live their dreams - and decided there and then that I had to live mine.

Four days after I arrived back home I had hatched many hair-brained schemes on how I'd become a business tycoon and self-made multi-millionaire, when the news came on in the background. I was sitting with Joanne discussing 'my incredible' ideas, as it was announced live that London had just won the 2012 Olympic bid! The crowds in London erupted at the news, and in my excitable state, so did I.

"Yessss, we've beaten the French" I shouted, punching the air in celebration, as I jumped off the couch in surprise! Joanne jumped up to, joining me as we danced around the living room like a pair of big kids. "There'll be a party in London tonight", she said, as the scenes of mass elation continued to be broadcast. "Yeah, what a great atmosphere for Sne and Mbali too" I said smiling.

Throughout the day the news swept the country and you could feel an excitement and energy in the air, brought on by this unexpected surprise.

By 8.51am the next morning the world had turned again. As I woke up I'd expected to see more coverage of London's Olympic triumph and the historic G8 conference being held at Gleneagles that day. Poverty was high on the agenda, as was increasing aid and writing off Africa's crippling debts.

But a new story was breaking this morning, and now being aired live on almost every channel.

I watched in stunned silence and the blood began to drain from my face. "What's up" Joanne enquired as she entered the room. I looked at her dazed, but didn't speak.

Horrific reports were coming in of a sequence of almost simultaneous suicide bombings across the capital. "Oh my God," I whispered. "I think Sne, Mbali and Hedwig are sightseeing in London today."

It is better to do well than say well

Magic and Madness

7th July 2005 and London was in the midst of its worst terrorist attack in history, which would end with fifty-two people dead, and over 700 more injured.

What twisted fate had brought Hedwig and the children here at this awful time I didn't know, but surely they haven't survived a lifetime of traumas just to be caught up in this madness. "They'll be OK, Kevin," Joanne said reassuringly as we watched the chaos unfold on the news.

Two days later and I received an email from the nuns telling me that Sne, Mbali and Hedwig were safe; the email was timed at 11.11 a.m., and I laughed as I surrendered my sanity to this peculiar phenomenon which wasn't going away.

As the year continued bizarre occurrences still happened to me daily, and I would continue to see repeat numbers everywhere I looked – such as 444 – and, more strangely now, I kept finding money on the floor everywhere I went.

I had become very philosophical about these occurrences, and having experienced events bordering on weird over the last few months, saw them as a good sign, as if fate was trying to point me in the right direction. But I still wasn't sure if I was simply in the middle of a midlife crisis, a spiritual transformation, or a complete mental breakdown.

Whatever was happening, it had been an unbelievable six months.

I had seen Sne in desperate trouble in February, only to have travelled an amazing journey of self-discovery to find him, before a strange twist of fate brought him to London, where we met again.

My family had moved from our small concrete prison of a house to an incredible home surrounded by large woodland gardens in April. These simultaneous events had allowed me to return to Zululand in early June, on another mind-blowing journey. This trip had culminated in food schemes being set up which would feed nearly a quarter of a million school meals of fruit to hungry children over the coming year, and set a string of other events in motion.

It was August now and we had just returned from a fabulous holiday of a lifetime in the Bahamas, where Joanne's sister had just married.

We'd spent two weeks all-inclusive on Paradise Island, Nassau, and my waistline was looking a little worse for wear. But I didn't care.

Life was good; no, it was better than good, it was amazing.

Yet deep inside me something was still missing.

I needed more from life now; I wanted to take control of my own destiny and live my dreams. I wanted to be able to go to bed each night satisfied that I hadn't wasted the day, but achieved something worthwhile, something that I had wanted to do.

But I wasn't sure what.

Joanne was enjoying our new lifestyle too. She hadn't said much about the fact I had committed to buying so much fruit when I had last returned from Africa, but she was slowly beginning to question my wisdom as our savings dwindled. She knew we needed a new car, and desperately wanted me to put some cash away for Rebecca and James.

On top of this my karate club was arranging a club holiday to Cuba in February and all our friends were going. Joanne wanted to go too, but I was reluctant to commit.

I'd been resisting Joanne on these financial fronts as I knew we needed to keep cash aside to pay for fruit each month and to travel back to Zululand in the future, but the issues kept coming up between us.

A few days after returning from holiday we attended a wedding party for friends and family who hadn't been able to make the trip to the Bahamas.

I was feeling tired that night and didn't want to drink, so decided to drive rather than take a taxi. It was late as we left the party and we had a half-hour drive back from Liverpool to the Wirral, a journey which requires the use of the Mersey tunnel.

As we approached the main tunnel entrance we discovered that it was closed for late night maintenance and we were redirected through a second tunnel.

"Damn," I thought as we exited the tunnel in an unfamiliar area.

"Do you know where we are?" I asked Joanne. She was tired and just wanted to get home to bed. "No, not really," she replied sleepily. "Follow the road, we'll soon find some road signs up ahead."

We drove for a few minutes, lost in unfamiliar surroundings, until unbeknown to me we entered a one-way system. As we did, another car was heading towards us erratically. As it came closer I realised it was in a one-way system and swerved in panic to avoid the other car.

The brakes screeched as I slammed them on and we hit the kerb at speed. I turned the wheel tightly to try and stop the car from crashing, but it was too late. The car mounted the kerb violently and hit a signpost so hard that it shot up in the air before rolling over on its side as it slammed back down to earth hard.

Adrenaline kicked in and time seemed to slow down. The noise was deafening as we crashed and I was left on my side looking at the floor, disoriented, and covered in debris. Joanne was screaming from the back of the car but I couldn't see what was happening; I managed to shift a little and turned and saw, despite her panic, she wasn't badly injured.

Rebecca was sitting next to me, dazed. "Don't move Bex," I said. "You'll be OK. Are you hurt?" She nodded to indicate she was okay. "Stay where you are, don't unbuckle your seatbelt or you'll fall on me." She nodded again and didn't move.

James had been sitting behind me in his child seat and I couldn't turn fully to see him.

"James!" I shouted. "James, are you OK?"

Joanne was still screaming, but James was deadly quiet and numbness struck me. "Oh God, no," I thought.

I managed to unbuckle my seatbelt and somehow managed to kick my way out of the window, and crawled out of the mangled car. Joanne was still screaming as I called James again. Tears were pouring down my face as I shouted again, but there was no reply. "James. James please…."

I dragged the passenger door open and looked at Joanne. I couldn't see James properly at first, but then saw he was still strapped to his seat motionless. I looked at him in sheer panic. "James," I cried. He turned slowly, looking back at me and pointing to his neck. "Oh God, you're alive."

"Are you OK, are you hurt?"

He didn't answer. He was dazed and confused and in shock, but Joanne managed to unbuckle him and I pulled him free from the car.

He was shaken up badly and had hurt his neck but he was OK. I hugged him like I've never held him before. "I thought I'd killed you," I said, shaking with emotion.

I quickly returned to the car and freed Rebecca. Then returned again and tried to free Joanne. A scene of chaos was developing around us as cars pulled up to help, and people ran from their houses to assist us.

Luckily, a police car had been travelling close by and seen the accident. Their siren was wailing loudly and the blue flash of their lights broke through the darkness of the night as they pulled up with a screech. Two policemen jumped out of the car and ran over to me to make sure the children and I were OK, before freeing Joanne from the car.

"You were lucky," said one of the officers as he spoke with me. His voice was trembling with adrenaline. "I thought we were coming to pull bodies from the car after the way we watched you crash."

A taxi driver ran up to us, his voice shaking as he spoke. "I saw the whole thing," he said to the policeman, before turning to me. "I can't believe you climbed out of that. There's someone up there looking down on you, son."

I looked at the car wreckage and a cold shiver ran through me. They were right. Ten beautiful nuns prayed for my family each day, and I had needed their prayers tonight.

We were taken to the police car to wait for an ambulance, which soon arrived and took Joanne and the children to the hospital for a check up, whilst I gave a brief statement to the police.

A few minutes after this, we set off to the hospital in the police car. We drove down a bypass onto the motorway and stared in shock as we saw my wrecked car being towed away; the wedding balloons we had brought from the party were flying out of the broken side windows, blowing happily in the wind as if in celebration of the night's events.

"You don't see that everyday," the officer said as we stared at the surreal sight. "No," I replied, laughing momentarily as I felt fate's hand at work once more.

I arrived at the hospital and was quickly reunited with my family. The car was a complete write-off, the signpost too – yet we had escaped with minor injuries of bumps, bruises and whiplash.

The next day we all woke up a little sore, but in relief that we were not badly injured or worse....

"What time is it?" I asked Joanne as I climbed out of bed. "It's time to thank your lucky stars," she said, smiling.

Later in the day I emailed Sister Hedwig, telling her of our brush with death and thanking her and the Sisters for their prayers!

email from Africa.......

Dear Kevin and Family...
I know God is great; he will never overlook the smallest kindness shown to his people to a thousand generations. That is why we Christians always say in God we store our future. We creatures sometimes want to see God's response to what we do and we do not see it and ask ourselves to what kind of person is God? God know best what and when we need it. So you have been labouring spending your money to come and help us and feeding 800 starving children at Palane, do you think God will forget that so easily? He won't. That is why he SAVED YOU and your family.
On behalf of the sisters, as delegated by the Sister Superior we say – Sorry to you and your family – we will continue to pray.

Having told me I was going to hell as a non-practicing Catholic on my previous visit, the sisters were now telling me their God had saved my life and my family!

I had never cared much for their prayers and knew they had better things to pray for than me. Besides, if there was a God up there looking after everything, why didn't he stop me from crashing in the first place, or feed the thousands of hungry children in Zululand, or the millions more around the world?

It didn't make any sense.

Hedwig had told me that God moved in ways we were not meant to understand, and that all things were his will. But I couldn't accept this blindly like she did.

Nevertheless, her email had made me realise that if I had died that night, nearly nine hundred children would no longer be fed each day…and I had to do something about that quickly.

The most amazing thing about the crash though was that it was almost as if it was supposed to have happened. Within a few weeks of the crash the insurance payout had paid for the new car we had been arguing about whether to buy or not. After paying for the car, enough money was left for us to go to Cuba with our friends as we had wanted to. And a little later, James and Rebecca each received compensation payments, and we finally had money to put away for their future.

We had wanted all these things, and the car crash had brought them all!

Best still, I hadn't had to spend a penny of the money I had set aside to feed the children in Nkandla.

As I realised the positive effects of the crash, I looked at Joanne and laughed. "Be careful what you wish for – you may just receive it!"

Joanne looked back, her eyes sparkling in wonder. "Yeah, you're right there," she said, smiling widely.

Every cloud has a silver lining

Food to Schools

Fifteen days after we got back from the Bahamas, and the resort we had stayed at was battered by a powerful tropical storm, which wreaked havoc. Four days later, and the storm had strengthened to become one of the most devastating hurricanes in history, Katrina, and slammed into New Orleans with winds and surging flood waters, which wiped the city off the map.

Climate related natural catastrophes had more than doubled in the last twenty years, and scientists had long been warning of the pending dangers of global warming. But economy and wealth was still more important than climate change to most of the world's politicians, and the Bush administration had pulled the US out of the Kyoto agreement four years earlier in 2001, destroying any chances of the world uniting to reduce global emissions.

Sadly, one of the areas which would be hardest hit first was Africa, and famine and death were destined to plague the continent for decades to come.

Whatever the future held, I knew I had to push on with my schemes and with the passing of each month, Phalane Primary School received about 18,000 school meals of fresh fruit for its hungry pupils; but I was becoming increasingly mindful that my savings were slowly diminishing.

Despite the fact my life was good, in the back of my mind my happiness was tinged with the knowledge that forgotten children were still left hungry, out of sight, out of mind, and I felt helpless to do more.

I was still searching for what I wanted to do with my life, and I wanted to find a way to link my personal ambitions with raising more money to feed more children. As I started to set new goals for myself I thought of the thousands of malnourished children in Nkandla still going hungry each day.

I knew there were easily five thousand kids there who needed food so I started playing with some sums. To feed five thousand kids a day at 4p a head was £200. Over a five-day school week that was £1,000 per week! A typical annual school term ran for forty weeks, so to achieve my goal I would need to raise £40,000 per annum.

I carried on analysing the unpleasantly large figures.

Okay, £40,000 would provide how many school meals a year; as I saw the number I dropped my calculator on the desk, "No, that can't be right" I mumbled in disbelief.

I picked up my calculator and started again. "No way, Joanne, come and look at this!" I shouted. At 4p a meal, forty thousand pounds would provide ONE MILLION school meals, feeding five thousand kids a day!!

"Wow – goal number one, raise forty grand," I said. No small feat, but not impossible either.

"How much is that each month?" Joanne asked inquisitively. "I don't know," I said as I divided my target by 12 months.

I sat staring into my calculator, speechless, as the numbers came up. It had been a typically annoying morning, and as usual I had seen repeat numbers everywhere. The last few days had become so bad I had started to remove clocks from sight as it was becoming annoying, but now I just stared into the calculator in utter disbelief.

"Well?" Joanne asked impatiently. I didn't speak as I passed her the calculator. Her eyes widened as she read the numbers: £3333.33. I looked at Joanne and didn't know whether to laugh or cry. I saw repeat numbers like this ten times a day, and as crazy as it sounds, I felt I was being told this is what I had to do now.

Everything you can imagine is real
Pablo Picasso

Maddening Burden

Sadly, when it came to fundraising I was a complete amateur.

I spoke with a couple of local Catholic schools about what I was doing in Africa and they kindly held events to help raise some money. My karate club got involved too, and during the next two months I raised about £500, which would pay for 12,500 meals. But these were single events and I needed an ongoing source of income, and I struggled to gain any momentum with my fundraising.

At the same time Sister Hedwig was still telling me disturbing stories of daily life in Nkandla, and email after email told of the horrors she was witnessing.

email from Africa.......

Dear Kevin...
... People are still dying as before even more now, especially young people. If one were to get used to death, then I would say we are used to it. People are dying. Wherever one goes there are lots of new graves and in many places they run short of grave yards. At Empapngeni they drive 18 – 22 km to bury their dead because of the lack of space.

Dear Kevin...
... One of my 9 year old boys in a family I help died. The father is sick he has TB. In addition to his sickness and the stress of having lost the 9 year old, he has to look after a 7 year old and a 4 year

old because their mother deserted them. It is painful to watch and hear what people go through here in South Africa... I hope it is not like this in other countries.

Dear Kevin...

... Many families are left only with children. I took quite a number of children to the Sizanani orphanage which is the mission place I run, but there is more need than space. I wish I could take them all but I cannot. Our government has a problem because it still puts restrictions to taking them to places like Sizanani even though there are so many left alone. Most of these children are hungry and sick. There are many children in Nkandla who die before their time and their deaths are not even registered most of the time.

With each painful email the clouds of despair grew bigger in my mind. I was desperate to help, but failing miserably.

I tried to raise grants and spent the next few months jumping through hoops and   getting nowhere. Some organisations refused to help with food aid; others didn't work outside the UK; others wouldn't help in South Africa; others only wanted to help specific schemes.

Those few who may be able to help needed me to apply as a registered charity, and then they would help only if the scheme was sustainable, ignoring the fact that children would die because of their red tape.

There's an old Chinese proverb "Give a man a fish and he will eat for a day. Teach him how to fish and he will eat for a lifetime."

This proverb had become the cornerstone of most funded projects. Yet sadly, at grass roots level, it was surprisingly and dangerously misleading, and ignored deeper problems.

Zululand was an area of hunger, yet in Natal there was no shortage of food. It grows so abundantly, in fact, that the area is known as the "Banana Belt" because of the millions of hectares of prime land which grow fruit there.

The problem was that the food got shipped off in the opposite direction to the ports and beyond. It was not given to the poor, or the sick, or to child orphans who were economically estranged.

Charities wanted schemes which would teach child orphans to fish, not to feed them with fish. How can you teach a young child to fish, when they are surrounded by poverty and if you gave them a fishing rod someone else would steal it from them? They wanted schemes where homeless orphans could grow vegetables – not accepting they had no plot of land to grow food on, no time or skills, nothing to cook with – and even if they could overcome all these obstacles and survive month after month waiting for the vegetables to grow, another hungry person would come and take their crop anyway.

You could raise money for a rape crisis centre to counsel raped children, but you couldn't raise money to prevent children from being raped. You could raise money to educate communities on how to grow food, but not to give them seed or to feed starving children facing death.

Common sense had been lost somewhere; love too.

I knew from experience the best way to empower the Zulu children was to educate them; the best way to educate them was to encourage them to attend school with food incentives. The food kept the children alive and removed them from begging and prostitution, improving their health and mental wellbeing as a result. All whilst providing vital trade with local fruit-sellers who desperately needed someone to sell their produce to.

These schemes would sustain an entire community. It took so little to do so much, yet no one seemed interested. My hand didn't fit their glove and that was that.

I tried to form a charity despite the obstacles, but was sent hundreds of pages of forms to complete…and the process was going to take six months to complete as a minimum. I just didn't know where to begin and had wasted too much time and effort chasing my tail already.

I felt responsible for helping these children, and I knew I was letting them down each day I failed to raise money to feed them.

My savings were steadily diminishing; they weren't a bottomless pit and wouldn't last forever. I needed to do something quickly to secure the schemes, but I didn't know what.

I'd been having sleepless nights for some time now, trying to dream up new ways of generating extra income. One night I lay in bed without sleeping at all, deep in worry for the children and what I should do next. I'd hit a dead end trying to fundraise and the press weren't interested in the plight of the children either.

If you walked into a school and killed a child, you'd be on every news bulletin and in every newspaper around the world – but if you tried to save thousands of children, the press simply didn't want to know – it just wasn't news.

I needed to find a steady income source if the feeding project at Phalane school was to be secured for the foreseeable future and I had to reassess my personal goals of trying to live my dreams.

Then, as if my magic, a few days later I was offered an additional part-time job, which I took and would work for the next 18 months, simply to earn 'banana' money to feed the children.

Half an egg is better than an empty shell

A Christmas Crisis

Christmas was approaching fast. I had been working my additional job a couple of months now and it had meant I was working another ten hours a week, which I didn't really mind.

In reality, two extra hours work a day secured enough money to feed and educate 886 impoverished children, and financing the project in this way made complete sense to me, even if it didn't to Joanne.

Only a few people knew I had taken the work on to feed a school in Zululand. I didn't even tell the nuns; there was no reason to. Besides I was a deeply private person and didn't want the world to know or judge my affairs.

I was more content now and sleeping better, knowing that the scheme was secure and would carry on into the future.

Joanne was a little worried that I was working too hard, but we'd had an amazing year and were both looking forward to a relaxing Christmas before our holiday to Cuba.

Sister Hedwig had been in frequent email contact with me, and I had been trying to get one of her sick brothers onto anti-retroviral drugs for about a month. She was resisting my offers as she was concerned the drugs could do him more harm than good in his deteriorating condition.

Sister knew I was trying hard to raise money to feed even more children, but she was content that the project at Phalane was going well and trusted in her God that things would happen when they should.

email from Africa.......

Dear Kevin...
... I appreciate the help towards my brother's treatment BUT I fear he is not too well and if he starts the treatment and defaults it, I might feel we have aggravated it with treatment...
...The project at Phalane goes well...Thank you for your sleepless nights trying to help...If God wants it to spread, they will help those who can, if not, then let us leave it to Him...

Hedwig's words reiterated her belief that everything that happened in the world was in God's hands.

I didn't see it that way. I had two hands of my own and believed that if we wanted something to happen, it was up to us to use them. Nevertheless her words eased my burden and I took comfort that I had provided nearly a hundred thousand school meals of fresh fruit to hungry children since June.

The more I reflected on Sister's words the more I felt mankind's hand seemed to do more harm than good most of the time. The UK was still fighting devastating wars in Afghanistan and Iraq, and soldiers and civilians alike were dying daily. Global warming was becoming indisputably a consequence of man's activities, yet politicians and powerful corporates still tried to grey over the matter to protect their 'interests'. The world had gone to pot and people didn't seem worried that children would die because of their actions, or inactions.

As Christmas approached, I was in need of a break. I had taken two weeks off work and wanted to relax for a few days before hitting the gym in my annual bid to get fit.

Christmas day was magical. Despite my experiences of poverty in Zululand I spoilt my children with gifts, and we ate and drank merrily, enjoying the peace and the time together.

We held a party on Boxing Day, and for the first time in many months, the awful plight of the Zulu children slipped my mind as I celebrated with family and friends.

By late evening I was happily drunk; yet for some reason decided to check my emails before I fell in to bed. "Ahh, there's an email from Hedwig" I said to myself as I logged on.

I opened the email, smiling, thinking it was a Christmas greeting from my friend from afar, but sobered up instantly as I read of her plight.......

email from Africa.......

Dear Kevin...
...It is hard for Sr Hedwig at times. My brother, the very same one you wanted to help is dying in hospital. It is so difficult for me to live with the anxiety and fear of hearing another striking news

after losing two other brothers but God knows and has a purpose for me I believe...

...I feel so tired and worn out...let me stop here for the day.

Merry Christmas

I typed back immediately.

Dear Sister...

...I am so sorry for your news. I can pay for AIDS drugs and send money tomorrow. If these drugs will save your brother, please let me know and I will send you the money straight away.

Hedwig's next email arrived three days later...

Dear Kevin...

... My brother struggled for some time trying to resist leaving us again after both parents and two brothers, but it seemed he could not escape it and he finally passed on.

"Damn it!" I shouted as I slammed the table hard with my fist. I'd been too late. I'd failed my friend; I could have and should have saved her brother.

"What is it?" Joanne asked anxiously. "Sister Hedwig's brother has died, I could have stopped it – he should have lived." I was angry. How could Sister Hedwig's God do this to her? She was an angel in my eyes who had given her whole life to his service, spending her days in worship and helping those in need. In return she was left to endure a living hell daily. Now, one by one, her God took her family and she was left believing they were to spend an afterlife in hell as non-practising Catholics!

I emailed Sister over the next month in a futile attempt to give her some words of comfort and support, but what could I say to someone with her beliefs?

I knew her brother's death must have torn at her soul, and surely made her question her steadfast belief that God had a master plan, or that he was just or fair.

Her brother's death destroyed me too. I knew I should have done more to save him, and I had failed. His death had left two more children orphaned, and I could have stopped this. Hedwig helped thousands of people and if I had supported her properly, then she would have remained capable of helping them.

Now she was lost to despair, and could help no one.

I thought I had grown spiritually since first travelling to Zululand, but like an unpredictable game of snakes and ladders, fell swiftly from the dizzy heights I had experienced, straight back down to the bottom of the board.

I knew no more now than I had known back in February when I lived happily in ignorance of the plight of others around me. My philosophical questioning of who I was and what life meant had seemingly taken me nowhere.

All too soon I returned to work and back to my part time job, and back to questioning my life. What was I supposed to be doing in life, where on earth was I heading?

When the night is darkest, the stars shine the brightest

Taking Control

It was early February and nearly twelve months since my life had been turned on its head by Sne's plight. I still hadn't heard from Hedwig and was beginning to feel isolated, working hard for children I was starting to disconnect with. Joanne was questioning why I was working so hard each day and wanted me to quit it and settle back into a normal life.

I vented some frustrations by training hard in the gym, and at martial arts, getting fit for our holiday to Cuba and trying to put Nkandla out of my mind.

Part of me yearned to travel back to Africa and help Hedwig in her time of need, but part of me wanted to move on, and focus on my own life once more.

Our second Caribbean holiday in six months was approaching fast, thanks to the extraordinary good fortune we were experiencing at the moment. A group of twenty-five of us were travelling to Cuba, and it would be a fourteen-day party of eating, drinking and having fun. Despite this temporary distraction in paradise, part of me was always somewhere else, somewhere in Zululand.

By the time I returned home from Cuba, Sister Hedwig was back in contact, and she was slowly recovering from her loss.

email from Africa.......

Dear Kevin...

...I am almost sure that you do understand what is going on with me now. All I can say is that I am still alive and kicking. Life seems to be hitting hard on me...

...We can do nothing to stop people from dying if that is how God has planned it. But what I strongly believe we can do, is to be there for those who are traumatised by the loss. To give emotional support, food since it is the main thing even for the sick to boost their immune system in order to live longer and take care of their own children. We can less the stress in children, I believe by sending them to school to be away from all these worries of watching their own parents dying in front of them because they cannot do anything about it.

...It is not only my brother dying, there are many people dying the same way by the same sickness – AIDS. It was almost a week after my third brother died and I was told my cousin died also...

Somehow Hedwig was slowly regaining her faith, but I had no such support mechanism. I was still struggling to live my daily life in my world of 'normality'. Sitting at work, or at home, I was constantly plagued by demons, knowing that if I just got up again, if I just took action now, I could save a child's life that very day.

This daily notion of saving the children was causing great conflict within me. Doing the right thing was not always easy, I knew that. But knowing the right way to do it was proving to be even harder.

I was beginning to lose my focus, when, thankfully, I was invited on a three month black belt course in martial arts. This subsequently extended over the next five months, stretching me to my physical, emotional and intellectual limits. Yet despite the immense intensity of this course, at its core was the key to learning to balance the three aspects which make us all human; the physical body, the emotional heart and the intellectual mind - and it helped me to regain some balance in my turbulent life.

As I rebalanced I knew I had to do more to help Hedwig and the forgotten children of Zululand. I wasn't one to go, cap-in-hand, begging for donations or help; aspects of my personality held me back from telling people of my efforts in Africa. I wanted to put something in place and wanted to live my dreams. If I could gain personal financial success, I could feed many, many more children this way.

My motivation to take responsibility for myself and live my dreams was growing stronger, and I started to put various ventures together, but ultimately none bore fruit quickly.

Through this time Sister Hedwig was still emailing me frequently with horror stories of what was happening on the ground in Nkandla, and these emails began to strengthen my resolve to succeed.

email from Africa.......

Dear Kevin...
....Recently I helped a 12 year old girl who had never been to

school. Her parents are dead and she lives with her grandmother who is very sick and her six year old cousin. They live on begging from neighbours or getting food from the convent...They live in a terrible place between mountains and forests as the only family. One night they heard some heavy footsteps around their old hut. The footprints, when looked at the next morning, showed to be that of a lion...

...we are moving them from there now.

As my martial arts course and demonstrations finally came to an end mid-September, I knew what was important in my life more than ever.

I knew I had to return to Africa.

Some people live their dreams, others seem asleep their whole lives

The Call of Africa

My trips to Africa were always the same: spontaneous, unplanned and a little upsetting for Joanne and my children.

Joanne had seen me working an extra part-time job for over a year now, and having just watched me train myself into the ground each day through martial arts, she wanted some 'us' time.

We had been planning to go on holiday in November for a week to spend some family time together; but Africa was calling me once more…and it was a call which was impossible for me to ignore.

Sister Hedwig's email was unpredictable. You could email her one day and receive a reply the next, or it could be weeks if not months before you heard from her. Her access to a computer was sporadic, and even when she had the opportunity to email me, I knew her computer was unreliable.

I contacted Sister, telling her that I would return in December, not knowing if she would receive my email. But a few days later I received an excited reply telling me of her delight and how she would arrange to pick me up at Durban airport for the long drive into Nkandla.

I had been monitoring late-deal travel websites for the cheapest airfares, and found some good flights leaving early December which gave me plenty of time to prepare for the trip ahead.

Joanne knew I had to return to Africa and was comforted by the knowledge that Sister Hedwig would be picking me up and taking me into Nkandla safely.

Over the next week I monitored the ticket prices for the best deals and decided I would soon set the date of travel and secure a ticket whilst they were cheap. This would give me plenty of opportunity to arrange time off work, and from my part-time job, whilst providing Joanne enough time to prepare for my departure and the inconveniences this would bring.

As the days passed, contentment grew within me once more, knowing that I would soon be helping the Zulu children again soon.

It was a cold Thursday morning in November and as the pelting rain bounced off my windscreen as I drove to work, I decided the time was right to book my ticket and return to Zululand.

I shot out of work at lunch time and came home to look for the best date with the cheapest flight. Joanne sat with me, keen to plan the dates which would suit her best too. We had looked at the prices only the night before and selected some good dates, but as I checked the prices again, they seemed to have doubled!

"What the...." I said as I tapped in the dates and looked at the astronomical prices. "Have you put in the wrong dates?" Joanne asked, looking at me and pulling a face to indicate my inept computer skills.

"Yeah, hold on, I'll do it again," I said as I reset the page and re-entered the dates. "No way, what's going on – the prices have more than doubled since last night."

Joanne was laughing, "That can't be right, watch out, I'll do it," she said, thinking I had messed it up again.

She re-entered the dates and we waited for a few seconds as the screen flashed and pulled up the prices. "You're right, they've gone right up," she said, shocked at the massive increase.

We looked at each other in puzzlement. "Kevin, you're trying to fly out in December which is peak summer time in South Africa, so they must have gone up to account for this and for Christmas holidaymakers," Joanne said.

I started to panic. The new prices were wiping out my travel budget and threatening the journey. "Try some other dates, there's got to be some cheap tickets left somewhere," I said.

We spent the next half-hour checking times and dates on various sites, but it was too late. The prices had risen overnight and that was that, I couldn't afford to travel in December and take enough money to make the trip worthwhile.

Joanne went to make a cup of tea to take a break. "I'll check some in November," I said. She looked at me with a menacing frown but said "OK. I'll be back in a minute to look with you."

Late November was the same as December. All the prices had

doubled and I couldn't afford to travel. I kept looking and as Joanne returned with the tea, I found a return ticket under the thousand-pounds-plus of the others.

Joanne sat down as I put my head in my hands. "What's up, can't you find any flights we can afford?"

I looked at her despairingly. "Just one," I said. "But I have to travel in 36 hours."

"Kevin, you can't....what am I going to do? I haven't got time to prepare for that."

I knew she was right. Leaving this quickly was going to cause her a lot of upset, the children too, and what about my lift from Hedwig, and time off work?

"If I don't book this ticket now I can't go before the new year. I have to go now, I know it's meant to be," I said in frustration.

Joanne was trying not to cry, but tears were welling in her eyes. I knew I was letting my family down again, but she turned to me and nodded, yes.

She had given me the go-ahead again, but I didn't know what to do; I sat in confusion for a moment, debating the situation in my head.

I didn't want to leave this quickly but I had to make a decision fast. I looked back at the screen as I searched my heart, then booked the ticket and it was done.

I was travelling Saturday morning and I was going to have to work rapidly to prepare for the journey.

Time and tide wait for no-one

God Speed

Everything felt wrong now; everything was rushed.

I quickly emailed Sister Hedwig with my new plans. I was leaving in 36 hours, but wouldn't land in Durban until the day after. Maybe there was still enough time for her to pick up my message and collect me from the airport.

A lift from the nuns was the safest way into Nkandla, and if Joanne knew I was being collected by the sisters she would feel a whole lot better about my journey and relax a little.

I needed to get some South African Rand too. I had no time to order any now and would have to act fast to get hold of small denomination notes. We had some second-hand children's clothes and toys my children had grown out of which I could take and it didn't matter if my case was a little light, I might be able to buy what I needed in Durban.

I had finished my part-time job for the day and would have to tell the boss tomorrow that I needed to shoot off for a week at short notice.

I spent the rest of the day making calls, buying supplies and organising my trip.

I woke in the morning feeling panic and the familiar feeling of pending danger that accompanied each of my trips into Zululand. It was going to be a long day, and as I headed out to see the boss of my part time job to tell him I needed some time off, I was feeling stressed.

I was paid on an hourly basis and only charged for hours I worked, so it shouldn't be a problem taking any time off. I'd worked into the late hours the previous night to finalise a work report and all I needed to do was speak with the boss and make some quick changes for him, then I could go without leaving any loose ends.

As I entered the office I found he was in a meeting and his day seemed to have started on the wrong foot with a number of unexpected business problems. I needed to speak with him quickly if I was to complete my report before I left, and perhaps leaving at such short notice wasn't going to be as easy as I had hoped.

I sat around for the next hour waiting patiently for him to free up, so I could speak with him and talk through the report. When he finally became free he was spitting feathers, angry with his problems of the day. Five minutes of his time was all I needed to get on with my work, but they were to prove a long five minutes.

"Hi, Trev," I said with a smile to easy the atmosphere a little. "Can I see you for a minute so I can finalise the report you need?" "I'll come and see you when I'm free," he replied abruptly as he marched out of the room.

I'd known Trevor for years and considered him more of a friend than a boss, but he was having a bad day and he would traditionally take it out on everyone else when he became this way.

When we finally got together we were like flame and fuel. He was stressed out with business and I was stressed out with life, and a row soon erupted.

To cut a long row short, I told him I needed time off work and he told me he wasn't happy about my attitude - as I told him I wasn't happy with his.

After a short unpleasant exchange of words, Trevor looked at me, barking "If you're not happy, why don't you leave then?"

By now, I'd had enough and was getting close to clocking him one. I stood up and looked at him blankly. "What a good idea," I wisped sarcastically, and with that picked up my coat and walked out.

I arrived home feeling like a great weight had been taken off my shoulders. I had only taken on the job over a year ago to feed children, and that had made it hard enough, and in truth I'd gained little satisfaction from the work whilst I'd been there.

In the beginning the work had been a godsend, helping me feed the children, but lately it had been causing friction at home and I had begun to feel stifled. As I arrived home I told Joanne of my row, and she was delighted at the news that I wouldn't be working the extra hours anymore.

"What about the school children in Phalane we are feeding?" Joanne said. "You'll have to tell the nuns you can't help them anymore now," she said as if probing my inner thoughts.

I knew some things were fated to happen and leaving the job had come at the right time, if not in the right way. "I don't know," I said. "Something will turn up, besides the job has been holding me back from helping the children more lately."

I felt happy now. I hadn't realised what a huge burden the extra work had been to me, and the relief of leaving it behind was instant.

I spent the rest of the afternoon rushing around preparing for my trip before spending time with Joanne, Rebecca and James.

Later in the evening the butterflies in my stomach were beginning to build, so I went to karate to blow off steam and burn off some pent up energy.

I didn't know it then, but tomorrow I would embark on another journey in Zululand, which was to prove even more incredible than my previous trips.

As one door closes, another door opens

Back to the Beginning

I woke in the morning feeling tired. I remembered how my first journey to Africa to search for Sne couldn't come fast enough, and how in contrast, this trip had been flung upon me so quickly I couldn't breathe.

I checked my emails expectantly, but Sister Hedwig had not been in contact. Had she seen my message yet? Would I get a lift, or would I have to struggle back in to Nkandla alone?

It was too late to worry now. I knew each time I walked into Zululand, magic happened, and as usual had no idea what lay ahead.

As the time to leave got closer there was an uneasy tension running through the house. Joanne had been agitated all morning. I knew she was angry at me for leaving so quickly. We had been considering going on holiday around this time, and she was having to make sacrifices for me once more. But she was consoled by that fact that if I took this journey, my simplest of actions could transform the lives of desperate children - and she knew I had to go.

James and Rebecca were upset too - James especially. He was unusually quiet so I tried to make a fuss of him before I left.

"What's up, little man?" I said to him, smiling, but he wouldn't look at me or talk to me. "What is it, what's wrong?"

James walked over to me slowly and sat on my knee glumly. "I want to keep you as my dad," he said sadly. "What do you mean?" I said, laughing. "I don't want you to leave me to be the dad of those other children."

I got a lump in my throat as he spoke and was desperately trying to hold back tears. James thought I was leaving him forever to stay in Africa to become the father to other children who needed me there.

"No, it's okay," I said quickly. "I'll be back in a few days. I'm not staying in Africa forever, I'll be back home to you very soon."

He was only seven and didn't understand, and wasn't convinced. He sloped off quietly to his room with his head low and I felt gutted. How could I have done this to my own son? He thought I was leaving forever and I would never return. I wanted to convince him I would be back soon, but I couldn't even guarantee him that. In the back of my mind I knew the journey held certain dangers and at any moment a cruel twist of fate could result in my death. I was breaking the heart of my children trying to help others in need and I couldn't justify my actions to them unless I returned safely.

I felt so angry for putting my family through this again and wanted to abandon my trip and stay home. What was I doing anyway? I despised travelling at the best of times, so why was I putting myself at risk again? My intentions had always been good, and in the beginning that seemed like enough. But would my own innocent children become fatherless through the folly of my actions? I was becoming agitated as the doorbell rang out loud and I knew it was time to leave. It was my brother Steve - he was driving me to the airport, and it was too late to cradle any doubts now. I would need my wits about me and would have to remain focused to survive the week and return safely.

Joanne, Rebecca and James came to wave me off, but it was a painful goodbye. James was grabbing my leg, crying, begging me not to leave him. Joanne pulled him away so I could go, but as I looked back at them through the car window as we drove away, I thought how it might be the last time they would see me alive.

It was an hour's drive to Manchester airport from my home. Steve was trying to make conversation, but I didn't want to talk. I was looking out of the window staring into space, thinking of James, and choking up at the thought I might die and never see him again.

It was a deeply depressing drive. I felt like a prisoner on death row being driven to my execution. My crime: stupidity; my punishment: death. It wasn't fair. I didn't want to die, not yet, not in the middle of Africa. I wanted to return to my family, and deep down wanted to stop the car and turn around and go home.

I arrived at the airport and tried to hide my feelings from Steve. He wished me well and I told him to look after my family, tormented by the thought that this could be a request lasting longer than the week.

I slowly wandered into the airport, feeling numb and nauseated, only to find an all-too-familiar scene of chaos. The London bombing were still fresh in everyone's minds and recently the UK had been put on another terrorist alert, warning of suicide bombers using liquid explosives to blow up planes in retaliation for the foreign wars Britain was engaged in with the US.

Enough dangers faced me ahead, but first I had to dodge religious men of faith who were still trying to kill randomly in the name of 'God'. We were living through a new era of religious tensions and a 'war on terror' had been declared.

I waited an age to check in my modest luggage before entering the departure lounge. As I passed the final checkpoint security staff demanded I hand over my bottle of water, deodorant and toothpaste - dangerous items which could all conceal explosives. I was heading back into hell to help forgotten children, and had no time for politically correct stupidity. I drank from the bottle to prove it wasn't going to blow up and sprayed myself down with the deodorant to display its contents, but it didn't matter.

People told me regularly that I was 'bananas', but I had learnt long ago that the rest of the world was far more crazy than me. Globally, we would allow a hundred and eighty thousand children to lose a parent to AIDS this month; leaving them to feel the grief, despair and fear I had first seen in Sne's eyes – yet the governments of the world didn't seem as interested in these children, as they did in my bottle of water.

"You smell very nice, Sir, but we're still going to need those items," the attendant said sarcastically. I reluctantly handed over my water and toiletries, shaking my head in contempt of the stupidity, as I passed through to departures.

By now my stomach was churning. Anger and apprehension always affected me this way before I travelled, and I headed quickly to the nearest toilets to relieve myself of my breakfast.

I settled a little after this, but as I was called for my first departure I knew the long journey was going to take its toll. My martial arts course had greatly improved my fitness, but it had come at a high price which was causing me much pain now. I had dislocated my shoulder three times this year already, once whilst I was training, and I had had to put it back in before continuing with the session. I'd also developed fallen arches, which was making it painful to walk. Worst of all I had a cracked disc in my back from another injury, which made it painful to sit confined for long periods of time.

I was last to board the plane, and as I passed through the luxurious large seats of first class, I sighed, and went to find my uncomfortable seat at the back of the plane.

As expected, the flights were tedious, tiring and painful. I couldn't sleep and spent most of my time wishing I was on a beach with my family, instead of here,   heading to Nkandla.

Despite the length of my journey my travel plans kept to schedule and I made all my connections without incident, wondering at each stage if Sister Hedwig had seen my email.

As I disembarked my final plane at Durban the warming summer heat hit with me a pleasant intensity, and I relaxed as my paranoid fears began to fade.

I was feeling fatigued, but the warming rays of the sun began to re-energise me as I remembered my previous journeys, and wondered what fate had in store for me now.

I stood waiting for my luggage, knowing the next half hour would shape the rest of my journey. I wasn't sure what I would do if Sister was not there to greet me as I left the airport. Would I try and drive to Nkandla or taxi in as I had in the past? Strange events always happened to me in this land of mystery and I smiled as I thought of bumping into David again, or perhaps someone new I was destined to meet.

As I walked out into the bustling airport I couldn't see any sign of Hedwig through the crowds. Then right in front of me a middle-aged white South African man turned around holding a makeshift cardboard sign, as he turned towards me I saw my name inked in large capital letters.

I approached the man and introduced myself, asking if he had been sent by Sister Hedwig. "Ah, so you are Kevin," said the man. "You have been causing much panic today. Sister Hedwig only read your email a few hours ago and has been running around the convent like a headless chicken trying to find a way to collect you." He was amused as he spoke and I could picture the scene of Hedwig's panic well.

"Sister Hedwig is on her way now and will collect you later. In the meantime you can stay at my house, or we can go shopping." "Thank you," I said, relieved, that Hedwig knew I was in the country.

As we made the ten-minute drive from the airport to his home we chatted politely about how I had first been drawn to Nkandla to find Sne, and of the many social problems facing South Africa. We soon arrived at his home and I was introduced to his family, who offered to take me shopping to kill some time. First I could take a shower and freshen up, a luxury I had not expected before my long drive into Natal.

My suitcase was lighter than usual because of my speedy departure and, as usual, fate seemed to intervene as if knowing a shopping trip was just what I'd hoped for. We soon headed to the packed mall and I spent the next few hours browsing the shops for bargain clothes, toys, medicines and sweets for the children I would soon meet.

I quickly found everything I needed before it was time to return to his home to wait for Hedwig. We had only been back at his house for five minutes, when there was a loud knock at the door. "Hello, Sister," said the man as he greeted Hedwig. "We collected Kevin for you safely as promised."

Sister entered the room wearing her familiar large smile. "Kevin," she said happily. "I only got your message this morning. We weren't expecting you for a few weeks yet!"

"Hi, Sister," I said as we hugged. "The plane ticket prices had skyrocketed and I had no choice but to book one quickly, or I wouldn't have been able to come at all."

I guess I had a strange relationship with Hedwig. She was a black Zulu by birth, and a converted Catholic nun by circumstance. Me, I was a white middle-aged married man with a couple of kids from Merseyside, who avoided church at all costs. Yet despite the fact I hadn't seen Sister since London, we were like old friends instantly.

We seemed bound by fate, having both felt the grief and suffering that the AIDS pandemic had brought to her people and, like her, I had vowed to do everything in my power to help the orphans left in its wake.

As we chatted, Sister introduced me to her designated driver for the day, a young volunteer working at the convent, called Deborah. "Hi, Deborah," I said, shaking her hand. "Hello, Banana Man," she said, laughing. "You are well known for what you do for the children in Nkandla," she said, smiling.

At home I was nobody special, and liked it that way. But in Nkandla I was fast becoming famous as 'Banana Man', to my continued embarrassment.

Courage without wisdom is foolishness

Death of Innocence

Sister chatted with her friends for a while before we decided it was time to head off on the long drive back to the convent.

I thanked the family for picking me up and taking me shopping, before collecting my luggage and preparing for the final leg of my journey.

"Kevin," said Hedwig as we climbed in the car. "We must first pick up a young lady from an orphanage to escort her back to Nkandla."

"She has had a terrible life and I have been hiding her away from Nkandla for over two years now because she witnessed her mother's murder. She has to return to give evidence in court in a few days' time against the men who murdered her parents."

There were over two million orphans in South Africa now, and each one had their own tragic story to tell. The children didn't just lose their parents here; they each lost their childhood, their innocence and any hope of a better future.

As we drove to the orphanage, Sister recounted the night of the murder with a level of trepidation in her voice.

"The young girl's mother was shot dead by the killers in front of her eyes, but she managed to escape from them. I had to find an urgent place of safety for her and her two-year-old cousin that night, and she couldn't even attend the funeral of her mother, as she was in hiding for fear the killers were hunting for her and her father.

"The father had escaped from them too. He came to me so I could arrange that he would take the children escorted by police, to hide them somewhere. The next day when he was supposed to be at my office, I received a call from the police to say he had been shot dead on the very same night he left me, his throat was cut open and they had nailed him to a tree before burning his hut to the ground.

"Because the girl was an eye-witness to her mother's death, the police used her to get information, so the killers are hunting for her. I have had to hide her far away in an orphanage. If we had kept her in the convent we would all have been in danger."

I could sense Hedwig's fear as she recalled her story. "I had to travel during the early hours of the morning and return at night," she said. "At least she is now safe, but she couldn't even attend the burial of her father either."

It had been over two years since the killings, but what shocked me most as Sister spoke was that it was not the first time I had been told this story. The very first night I had visited Nkandla the nuns had told me of this girl's plight and I had wished then that I could have been there to help the girl. Now, having been flung into travelling weeks earlier than I had planned, I would not only meet, but escort this very same girl back into Nkandla.

We continued to drive in the heat and humidity of the afternoon sun for about an hour, but I was drained after my journey and I was trying hard not to drift into sleep.

Sister had hidden the girl well. So well in fact, we seemed to struggle to find the orphanage for a while, but eventually we did.

As the car pulled up I looked at the surroundings of the impoverished orphanage in anguish. To walk into an orphanage such as this is heartbreaking. The children there were like rag dolls. They wore rag doll clothes, were housed in rag doll shelters and endured rag doll lives. Yet these were the lucky ones who had been taken in, away from the streets.

They had each lost their parents and had nothing in the world now but the clothes on their backs and each other. I wanted to hug each of the young children and tell them that everything would be OK, but it would have been a lie. Each had lost their childhood a long time ago and faced an uncertain future of poverty, hardship and pain.

Hedwig soon found her young orphan who, despite her environment, was sad to be torn from her makeshift family of friends; even in a place like this children could still find a smile, and a love in their hearts which was overwhelming to witness.

As we collected our young passenger and left for the convent, Hedwig was beginning to get hungry. I knew from our previous encounters Sister's favourite pastime was eating, and we faced a four-hour drive yet, so we decided to get some food before we left. We headed into a town and stopped off at a Kentucky Fried Chicken outlet, probably the first treat this young lady had received since being cruelly orphaned by the murder of her family.

After a short meal we returned to the car and drove and drove.

By now tiredness was overwhelming me and I struggled to fight off fatigue as the warm sun streamed into the car, relentlessly relaxing me. Each time I drifted off for a second, the bumpy roads would rudely jolt me awake, to the constant amusement of Hedwig and the others.

As the hours passed, my determination to stay awake steadily dissolved and sleep finally befell me. I woke sometime later, dehydrated and disorientated.

"How long have I been out?" I asked Deborah as I came around, rubbing my eyes. "I'm not sure," she said, "but I think your snoring put our friends back there to sleep too." I turned around and found Hedwig and the young girl flat out asleep. Deborah looked tired herself. She had been driving in the heat for nearly eight hours already today, and still had another two-hour drive or so before we would be at the convent.

I hadn't met Deborah before. She was from Germany, and as my head cleared, we chatted a little about what had drawn us both to help the children here. Soon Hedwig woke and as we got closer to the convent I started to gain my bearings.

"There's a fruit market over that hill, isn't there?" I asked Hedwig. "No, I think it's a little further on over the next one," she replied, trying to find landmarks as she looked. "Can we stop there to stretch our legs a little and buy some fruit?" I asked excitedly.

"Of course we can, Banana Man," laughed Hedwig, knowing my intention was to fill her car with as much fruit as would fit.

As we reached the market stalls memories of previous trips flooded back in. It took so very little to make such a big impact in this land of need, yet for reasons beyond my comprehension, few people seemed to help here.

As we pulled up to the market Hedwig got out of the car and followed me as the others climbed out to stretch their legs. As the traders saw us approach their excitement grew and they heckled us desperately to buy from them.

I bought as much fruit as I could from each trader and loaded the car with Hedwig's help. The car was soon full of the sweet smell of exotic fruits, and the traders' pockets were quickly full of money; so we set off slowly, looking for children to feed.

As we travelled we fed child after child, and humbleness engulfed me as it had so many times before. Sister laughed, as hungry faces appeared time and again to receive the much-welcomed food we were passing out. The final leg of the journey was filled with happiness as smile after smile thanked me for nothing more than an apple or orange or banana.

Despite the amount I had purchased, the fruit went quickly as we fed many hungry mouths in no time at all. Deborah seemed glad when the fruit was finally gone, and speeded up in a final push for home.

Darkness was falling as we reached Nkandla town and it was time we found sanctuary within the confines of the convent.

There was a small two-pump gas station on the verge of town and Hedwig asked Deborah to pull over and refuel the car for the next day.

"Is that wise with our young passenger here?" I asked Hedwig, a little concerned. "It will only take a minute," said Hedwig, "we'll be at the convent soon."

As we pulled up towards the pump, a car suddenly screeched up in front of us to block our way. Deborah hit the brakes hard to stop, as the unfriendly occupants of the car faced us down. It was obvious they didn't want any gas, and I looked at Deborah wondering why these idiots had blocked our path.

As we sat there another vehicle pulled up besides us, containing about twelve men in the back of a truck, who quickly started heckling Hedwig in native Zulu.

I didn't know what they were saying, but from the angry retorts of Hedwig it obviously wasn't pleasant. The men were laughing loud at first, but soon began to whip themselves up into an increasingly frightening frenzy.

I was beginning to worry whether they had noticed the girl in the back of our car, or were part of the gang who had killed her parents, when one of the occupants in the car in front of us climbed out and stood in front of his car menacingly.

I still couldn't tell what the truck full of men were shouting about, but began to get the uneasy impression they were making sexual threats against Hedwig and the others, and the situation was beginning to deteriorate rapidly.

Another car pulled behind us and we were blocked in on three sides now and going nowhere. I had left home feeling I would die during this trip and realised this could be that fatal moment.

Adrenaline kicked in and as it pumped through my veins my years of martial arts training allowed me to harness the enhanced powers this brought. My mental and physical responses had sped up by now. The movements and words of others had slowed down.

I had come here to save dying children with a pureness of purpose, but this mission deserted me as the dark mood of the moment swept in.

I couldn't stop all these men alone, but they weren't going to harm the girl, Hedwig or Deborah either while I still had fight in me.

I had unbuckled my seatbelt unnoticed and adjusted my posture so that it was light and agile, ready to exit the car rapidly. My left hand was on the car door handle and I was ready to pounce when the moment came.

The men in the truck to the right of me were still shouting abuse at Hedwig, who was angrily arguing with them and holding her own. The talk was in Zulu, but I knew the intentions here were bad, as the intensity of their words escalated.

The hairs of the back of my neck were standing on end now, not with fear, but with the powerful energies which were consuming me.

I was smiling coldly at the man standing in front of me. He was a young, tall Zulu and my reaction to him, and the situation around us, seemed to confuse him a little.

He started to walk slowly towards me and I watched each step, knowing his fate came closer with each one he took. His friend had remained in the car and looked like he was cradling a weapon, and I knew I would have to deal with them both quickly when the moment arrived.

Then my chest exploded.

It was if my very aura had ignited with emotional energy and erupted outwards like a volcano. Whatever energies powered my body, they were streaming out of me now with an incredible intensity.

I would likely be dead before this scene had played out, but this feeling just flamed the firestorm about to burst out of me.

I knew the exact distance at which I would have to exit the car and stop the man dead. He had paused one small step before this, and whilst consciously I didn't want him to move, part of me was begging for him to do so.

I had already visualised his death in my mind's eye, and knew exactly how I was going to kill him; it would take only a split second and I knew as he fell I would be able to reach his cowardly companion before he could get out of the car to brandish his weapon. The men in the truck were too distracted by the women sitting in the car with me, a deadly mistake which would cost them there lives this dark night...

The man in front of me had noticed my demeanour as I continued to smile at him menacingly with intent in my eyes. He smiled back nervously, but didn't take the fatal step. "Come on, you bastard," I said to myself as I beckoned him forward, "just one more step, just one more small step".

Time was running in slow motion now except for the energy bursting though my body, which seemed timeless. My mind was focused on everything, seeing everything, hearing everything. Nothing moved unnoticed. Whatever powers were in play now, they seemed to have stopped the man in his tracks a step short of his death.

The silence was deafening as a long stand-off ensued, then without warning the truck's engine next to us spluttered into life, and the gang drove off into the night, still hurling abuse at Hedwig, who was responding in kind.

As it pulled away my eyes continued to pierce through the coward in front of me, and his spineless friend who had remained in the car. He stood there a few seconds longer, unsure what to do, before turning away as he quickly jumped in his car which reversed out of the gas station and drove away beeping its horn.

The intense electricity of the situation could still be felt in the car and Deborah's sigh of relief pounded in my ears, as the standoff ended without incident.

I turned and looked at her but couldn't speak, as I tried to control my adrenaline gland and slow my breathing. She knew me only as a man of compassion, not one of destruction. But power is power… and the reality was I was a formidable obstacle to any who wished me harm. I was trying desperately to disguise my demeanour and disperse the adrenaline flooding through my veins, as I let the red mist of madness which had consumed me fade away slowly.

I don't remember the few minutes' drive back to the safety of the convent, but felt a great veil of shame fall over me as we drove through the gates. I had come here to save lives – yet had just come close to taking them away.

Anger restrained is wisdom gained

Calm in the Convent

The nuns were delighted to see us all safe as we entered the convent and they greeted us warmly. None of us spoke of the situation that had developed in town, and I tried to put it out of my mind as my senses returned to normal.

The Sisters had prepared a meal for us, and as Hedwig took her young guest to her room to settle her in for the night, I sat and talked with the others as I ate.

I hadn't seen the nuns for some time, yet as we talked it felt like I had never been away. Familiar cans of Castle Beer soon appeared on the table, something I needed after the tense standoff only moments ago.

"Kevin, you always surprise us with your visits," said Sister Ellen. "I was in the convent this morning when I heard Sister Hedwig running around shouting that you were arriving today. We weren't expecting you for a few weeks yet."

I had relaxed a little by now and laughed, knowing how I usually just turned up out of the blue, caused chaos in the convent for a few days, fed lots of hungry children, then disappeared as quickly as I arrived.

"I know," I said. "I had to get a ticket quickly as they had begun to increase in price for the winter sun-seekers trying to escape for Christmas. If I hadn't come now, I may not have been able to travel until February or March next year."

"You're an extraordinary man," said Sister Michaelis as she handed me another can of beer. I shook my head in disagreement, smiling politely.

It was the second time I had been called an extraordinary man by a nun, but I held the view that it was ordinary to feed children in need, and extraordinary not to!

But then I'd watched Live 8 come and go this year, the World G8 Summit in Scotland too – yet nothing had changed here on the ground. Actions speak louder than words, that was for sure.

We continued to talk and I remembered how the nuns had believed I was heaven sent on my first visit. Thankfully, now I had been downgraded to a Good Samaritan, something that I felt far more comfortable with.

I knew I wasn't the man they thought I was, but it gave them reassurance that someone somewhere was trying to help them, and if this gave them hope, then that was all that mattered.

Sister Hedwig walked into the canteen, smiling, and took a plate of food before joining us. "It's been a long day, hey," I said, smiling. "Yes," she said before tucking into her meal.

On my previous visits I had always been full of energy, but tonight I was exhausted and struggling to stay awake.

I had so many questions for the nuns - what was happening on the ground now, was anyone else helping, what was needed most here? But my questions would have to wait until I recovered.

I needed to catch up on some sleep if I was to survive the next few days.

I bade the nuns goodnight and dragged myself wearily to the guest house, which the Sisters had once again prepared for me.

I fell into bed, exhausted, and didn't wake for the next ten hours.

Face of the Future

The next morning I was awakened by the bright sun as it streamed through the thin curtains which failed to hold back its brilliance.

My head was still foggy with sleep after my tiring journey but I could hear people milling about outside and knew I had slept in too long. I was here for a purpose, not for a holiday.

I slowly got up and dressed, and wandered through the courtyard to find Hedwig and the others.

In the canteen Sisters Raphael and Colette were sipping tea, and they smiled warmly as I joined them for a cup to quench my thirst.

"Good morning, Kevin," said Raphael, almost in song. She was a young Zulu nun whose smile was constantly radiant, as happiness flowed from her and spread outwards.

Hedwig entered the room and joined us. "Hello, Kevin," she smiled. "Sadly I must work in the hospital today, but you can drive a car and take two local care workers who are going on home-based visits this morning."

"Oh, I'm not too sure it's a good idea for me to drive," I said nervously at the thought of navigating the narrow roads through the hillsides and valleys.

"That's OK," sister laughed. "We have another guest here who may be willing to drive. His name is Sidney and I'll go and find him and see if he will join you. If you wait outside at 11am, you can all meet by the white car and I will introduce you to each other."

"Okay," I said, relieved, and continued sipping my tea as Hedwig left to find Sidney and the others.

It was already 10.30am and I wasn't in the mood to eat breakfast, so finished my tea and returned to the guest house to empty my case and find some of the clothes and toys I had brought to hand out.

By the time I had returned to the car Hedwig was already waiting, chatting happily with the two care workers and Sidney.

"Hello, everyone," I said as I approached. "Hello, Banana Man," replied Sidney. "I've heard all about you - what an incredible story!" I lowered by head in reluctant acknowledgement, knowing I wasn't going to shake off my nickname no matter how hard I tried.

We chatted for a while, then Sister turned to us sadly, "I have to go back to work now. Sidney can drive and my colleagues will guide you to the families you are visiting." I looked at the two small white cars to see which one we were taking, then looked to the heavens, unfazed by the registration plates, which could only have ever been what they were - NKA 333 and NKA 222.

"Are you coming?" asked Sidney as he noticed my distraction. "Yes, but can we stop off at the market to buy some fruit?" I asked as we jumped in the car. "Sure," he said, as he turned the engine over a few times before it coughed into life.

We drove to market and I bought huge bags of oranges and bag after bag of bananas to hand out to the people we would meet as we travelled.

The care workers couldn't speak much English, and Sidney only a little Zulu, but between them they soon found the route to our first family visit.

It was a hot day and I chatted with Sidney as we drove. He was a Catholic who had come here to help the Sisters in their work. He seemed to understand the social position of the country better than anyone I had met before. Although he was South African, like me he couldn't understand how his countrymen, the government, or the wider world could stand by and leave these people to their terrible fate.

"Is it like this across South Africa?" I asked Sidney. "Worse in some places," he said with a tone of defeat. "Nkandla has the worst rate of HIV anywhere in South Africa, and a higher rate of poverty, but at least it still holds its rural traditions and natural beauty. In places like Cape Town and Johannesburg there are huge shanty towns, and they are dreadful places of squalor and breeding grounds for crime and violence."

"I know," I said. "South Africa seems to have a big crime problem." Sidney looked at me, resigned to this fact. "It always will have whilst 90% of people live in desperate poverty, while three million others hold all the wealth."

Sidney continued and the stark statistics were sickening. Over five and a half million people were suffering from AIDS in South Africa, mostly blacks without access to anti-retroviral drugs. A thousand people a day died of AIDS, leaving behind frightened orphans to a dreadful life of unnecessary suffering.

It was easy to get lost in the social problems of South Africa. It had a long and violent history ever since the Boers and the British invaded in the nineteenth century in a land grab. Discord escalated through Apartheid from the 1950s onwards until the turbulent 1980s, which saw years of unrest until the end of the decade when the abolition of Apartheid began.

Since that time the ANC government which had swept to power had done precious little to help its people inflicted by the AIDS pandemic, and a new elite group had sadly evolved.

South Africa was indeed plagued by horrific crimes, but you had to question just who was committing them.

We travelled a little further and soon found the homestead of our first family. We stopped as close as we could and climbed out of the car to walk the final distance, but at first there was no sign of the young mother we had come to visit.

The care workers asked some of the children where she was and we found her ill on the floor of her hut. She, like many in the area, had HIV, and she was pregnant and very sick.

She slowly sat up and the care workers chatted with her to assess her condition.

She was tired and looked drawn and didn't want to talk at first, but soon began to chat as she told us how her husband had left her to look for work in Dundee to help feed the family. She was upset and obviously ill and the care workers feared she may be losing her baby.

Her young daughter toddled into the hut and I greeted her with a big smile and gave her a soft teddy I had brought. She was shy at first but soon took the bear and grasped it tightly in glee. Sidney told the mother that I was helping feed the children at the local school and she seemed delighted.

"Two of her children attend that school," said Sidney. "She is very happy they are getting food there. She said her young daughter who you just gave the teddy to was crying this morning though, because she was too young for school and wanted to go there for something to eat."

I looked at the poor child and could barely contain my tears behind my sunglasses. I had set up food schemes to help children like this young girl, but today I had caused this child to cry with hunger because she couldn't eat whilst her brothers could! "What's up?" asked Sydney. "Nothing," I said, remembering the food we had brought. "I'm just going to the car."

I was angry now, with myself, with the situation, with this stupid crazy world.

I picked up as much food as I could carry and struggled back to the huts. "Tell her this is for her children," I said as I met Sidney outside the hut. "Save some for later," he said, knowing there was plenty of hunger in this land of sorrow. "I'll buy more later," I replied bluntly, still angry at the plight of the innocent child that my actions had caused to cry, only that morning.

I stomped back and forth to the car for supplies for the next few minutes and provided the mother with much food and medicines, as well as clothes and toys for her children, as she sat stunned by my actions.

As we were leaving I gave the lady a handful of money – which prompted Sidney to take out his wallet and do the same.

"A little money goes a long way here," said Sidney as we walked back to the car and I nodded knowingly. "How much did you give her?" he asked. "I haven't got a clue," I answered, and he smiled with amusement, knowing I had just given this lady a small fortune in an act of angry generosity.

I'd vented some frustration here. But the day was just beginning…

You can't change the past, but you can change the future

Orphans of Nkandla

We returned to the car and I began to lighten up a little as we drove. Sidney had been trying to come up with solutions to alleviate poverty and injustice in South Africa for decades. And I think today he had glimpsed the simplest way.

It was now left to individuals to turn the tidal wave of misery – and small acts of kindness at grass roots level changed lives beyond measure.

We continued driving and one of the social workers struggled with her English as she explained the typically tragic plight of the next family of children we would meet.

"Four orphans were left homeless after both parents died of AIDS," she said. "Their uncle took them in for a short while, but he was mentally ill and soon chased them away, leaving them completely homeless."

"The youngest orphan is only four, and the eldest is sixteen and is pregnant now with her boyfriend's child."

"That's awful," I said as anger began to build once more. "Are they still living rough?" "No, thankfully a kind old couple have taken them in and allowed them free use of a hut," said the lady. "We're going there now with some food parcels as the couple struggle to feed their extended family."

The midday heat was peaking as we drove further and further through the valleys to find the family. Finally we pulled off road, as the workers hoped they had tracked them down. "This way, we think," they called as they walked ahead to see if they had reached their destination. "Yes, we are here."

I helped Sidney carry food parcels from the car and we quickly followed the ladies to find the children. As we entered the homestead we saw three deprived children meandering around the huts. "Hello there," I said, smiling. They smiled back shyly before running off to hide.

The care workers were looking for Petros and Irene, the kind couple who had taken the children in. Soon, Petros appeared and welcomed us with a wide smile. He couldn't speak English and spoke in Zulu with the care workers and Sidney as they established how the young children were coping.

Sidney interpreted as they spoke. "Phiadlle, the eldest girl, who is pregnant, has gone to try and get a grant to help the children," he explained. "The children we met a moment ago are her brothers and sister and they have to sleep on the bare floor at night as the family is so poor they can't even afford blankets."

"What?" I said. "That's terrible."

Sidney looked at me sadly. "I know. It's like this across South Africa now," he said despairingly. "Petros and his wife do all they can to feed the children, but they are poor and struggle to keep them."

Despite his situation, Petros had a huge heart of gold, and disregarding the language barriers, we were soon laughing and joking together, as he played out funny scenes to explain his thoughts.

Petros had nothing in the world, yet he had found happiness in his humbleness, a rare quality that was deeply inspiring. He was a king amongst men; he had so very little yet shared it all: his home, his food, his happiness, his love – he shared them all with the desperate children who had arrived at his door.

I'm never quite sure what I am supposed to do when I come to Nkandla, into a land unknown, yet purpose quickly finds me each time I do.

"Why can't these children go to school?" I asked Sidney. "They can't afford the uniform or the fees," he replied.

In this land of death and despair the government made children pay to go to school, and insisted they wore a uniform! "If one were cynical they would say it was to keep the school numbers down – and therefore the costs," said Sidney, shaking his head.

"Tell them I will speak with Hedwig later and arrange money for the uniforms and fees," I said, knowing the only chance these kids had of a better future was through an education that could empower them to improve their lot.

The care workers said they thought Hedwig was already arranging for the children to go to school next term, but they told Petros anyway, and he shook my hand energetically, as a great shame swelled within me once more.

As usual I had brought toys, clothes and sweets and quickly passed them out to the children, who by now were far less wary of me. The joy this act brings to young faces is the same each time, and if you experience nothing else in life, these memories live with you forever.

Petros wanted sweets too, and had been eyeing up my England cap for some time by now. I passed it to him to try on and he ran off laughing, chasing the children and waving his prize in the air.

It was my favourite cap, but I should have known I'd lose it at some point. Each time I came here someone would pinch my cap sooner or later, and I was delighted this one would be treasured by Petros from this day to his last.

Soon it was time to leave, and I handed Petros a large wad of cash. I looked at him, smiling, and indicated it was for the children, and the happiness in his eyes thanked me deeply, but I wanted him to stop.

You never feel generous in these situations, just a mix of deep humbleness and despair, for being able to do so little, when so much is needed.

I looked at Sidney as we walked back to the car. "Can we buy blankets in Nkandla town?" I asked. "Yes, I think so" he said. "Can we head there now and return here later with some for the children?"

I continued.

"I don't think that's a good idea, despite your good intentions," he replied, to my surprise. "Speak with Sister Hedwig later. It may be better you return with her tomorrow so she can assess the condition of the children and produce a report. You can give them some blankets tomorrow."

"That way she will understand the children's needs and will be better able to help them in the future, so let's leave it for today." I looked at him, a little confused. "Sidney, it's not you who has to sleep rough on the floor tonight."

He seemed a little embarrassed to reject my request, but it was late afternoon and he wanted to return to the convent to rest, so we made our way slowly back, passing out fruit as we travelled.

We arrived back at the convent and dropped off the care workers before Sidney went to find something to eat. I wasn't hungry – how could I eat in this land of hunger? So I went back to my guest house determined to return to the children the following day with the best blankets money could buy!

By evening I was starving. I'd eaten nothing all day. I hated eating when I knew children around me needed the food more than me, but the compulsion to eat eventually won and I finally went to find the nuns.

I soon found Hedwig, Sidney and the others chatting about the day's events. "I hear you want to return to see Petros tomorrow," said Hedwig. "Yes, the children need blankets," I said. "They have to sleep on the floor."

"I will take you myself tomorrow," smiled Hedwig, and my mood changed to one of delight.

For the rest of the evening we sat around chatting, and I ate little, but drank lots. I still hadn't recovered from the inbound journey and was feeling tired, when a huge bang rang through the convent, followed by an intense flash of lightning.

The lights were flickering and the nuns went to fetch some candles. "You'd better head back to the guest house," said Hedwig. "These thunderstorms are very dangerous and could take out the power at any moment. In Nkandla, when there is lightning, people often die as they have little shelter."

I looked out of the window as the clouds formed and the heavens opened. I turned to Sidney, knowing we should have returned earlier to the orphans with the blankets, as they were now huddling on a cold bare floor, frightened and wet.

Live the moment

Butterfly Effect

The summer thunderstorm continued long into the night, but by morning the sun was burning hot once more.

I arose for breakfast and went to find Hedwig; I wanted to go to market early for provisions, before heading out with the blankets for the children, who must have endured an awful night at best.

I met Hedwig in the dining area and she beckoned me to sit and eat something before we set off, which I did reluctantly.

I hadn't had the pleasure of Hedwig's driving skills for some time, but as we left the convent, fear soon gripped me again as we hurtled towards anyone brave enough to walk in her way!

We entered the bustle of the market to the heckles of the traders, keen to do business. "Over here," Hedwig called, and I walked to one of the traders she knew. Within less than a minute we had cleared the lady's stall, and she sat in stunned silence as we packed our car full of her produce.

"Tell her she can take the rest of the day off," I joked to Hedwig who was by now used to my extravagant shopping habits.

Then I turned to Hedwig purposefully. "Where can we get blankets?" I asked. "There is a shop over here which should sell them," she said, and I followed her eagerly.

The price of goods in Nkandla is cheap and I soon found the thickest, softest, most expensive blankets the shop had to offer and bought four. They were more like mattresses than normal blankets, and as I struggled out of the shop with them, I knew the kids were going to love them.

We returned to the car and set off to find the Petros homestead, chatting happily and feeding children along the route as we travelled.

"Sister, the young children Petros looks after don't go to school at the moment," I said anxiously. "The care workers said you were trying to help them so they can go next term". "Yes," said Hedwig. "I am seeing to it that they can attend school soon, it is so important that they go."

"I know," I said, relieved at the news.

As we arrived we pulled off the track and parked a little way from the homestead. Sister beeped the car horn and two of the children came running to greet her, smiling and waving.

"We have some presents for you," said sister to the children as she struggled to pull the large bundle of blankets from the back of the car. The children's faces lit up with delight - and so did mine. No matter what else happened now, the sacrifices and dangers of the trip had been justified a hundredfold.

On my journey out I had wished I had been heading to a quiet beach with my family instead of here; but not now. To have found these children sleeping on the dirt floor and to have provided them with blankets, was to change their world, and this feeling was to live a lifetime of purpose in a single moment.

They grabbed a large blanket each and slowly struggled back to their hut, talking gleefully between themselves as they walked.

"I'll carry the other blankets, Sister, if you can bring some of the food." Hedwig nodded and we made our way to the homestead.

By now Petros and his wife Irene had heard the commotion and had come to see what was going on.

"Tell Petros I've come back for my England cap," I said to Hedwig. She relayed my message and a sad confused look washed across his face. I was struggling not to smile as I stared at him sternly, before bursting out into fits of laughter.

A large smile spread across Petros face as he suddenly realised I was pulling his leg, and we were quickly welcomed into his hut. Hedwig explained we had brought the children blankets after learning they had none yesterday, and she chatted about the children's health whilst I passed out sweets and played ball with the youngest. I couldn't understand much of what was being said until Petros pointed at me laughing loudly and declared 'Banana Man' as Hedwig told him how I was feeding many children through the school projects. I put my hand over my face and shook my head briefly in embarrassment, then looked back and Petros and started laughing with him.

The warmth and happiness of Petros could humble the soul of the coldest heart, and I felt privileged to have met him once more, before we said goodbye and left his homestead.

As we drove away I felt energised and happy, my soul full of purpose again.

Although Sister was with me, she had work to do that day, and desperately needed to find a young mother in the mountains, whose son was very sick and needed to attend hospital urgently for an operation.

"I am not sure where the mother is," said Hedwig, worried for the child. "He needs to go to hospital, but can't unless his mother agrees to sign permission papers."

We drove deep into the countryside, and the natural beauty of the area was as breathtaking now as it had been the first time I had witnessed it. As we travelled, Sister stopped regularly at the roadside, asking directions from locals who might be able to guide us closer to the family's home. Each time we stopped I passed out fruit to the grateful recipients, and would get out of the car to feed children as Hedwig talked.

We seemed to be heading in the right direction and soon found the area where the family might live. Mist clouds were forming over the mountaintops and the sight, touch and feel of the landscape was invigorating.

We left the roads and headed along bumpy dirt tracks, not knowing our final destination. We asked more locals for directions, but had hit a dead end in our search for the mother and child. We were just about to turn back when Hedwig saw a woman in the distance and beeped her horn. The lady approached us apprehensively, before speaking with Hedwig in Zulu for a while. "She thinks the mother we are looking for may live in a hut close by. She is going to see if she can find her, so we will wait here for five minutes to see."

We waited and waited, until finally a lady appeared in the distance and began to approach us. "This could be her now," said Hedwig, who had been growing impatient, and she drove slowly towards the woman and wound down the car window.

They spoke in Zulu for a time, but Hedwig was beginning to get uncharacteristically angry and her voice was rising. "What is it, Sister?" I asked with concern. Hedwig turned to me in annoyance. "This is the lady I have been looking for, but she is refusing to sign the permission forms for her son to have the operation to save his leg. If he doesn't have the operation he may lose his leg." I sat stunned for a second and looked down at my legs, then back at Hedwig.

"Why won't she sign the forms?" I asked, still confused at the situation. Hedwig spoke with her again to find out, then looked at me and sighed. "She can't afford the taxi-ride to the hospital and has no other way of getting there with her son." "How much does she need?" I queried. "About ten Rand."

"Ten Rand!" I was shocked at the drama which was unfolding around me. Ten Rand was about eighty pence, and feeling numb, I put my hand in my pocket and pulled out a large wad of ten Rand notes and handed them through the car window to the woman.

The mother's face lit up and her mood changed immediately, and so did Hedwig's. She quickly agreed to sign the forms and Hedwig was delighted that the child's leg would be saved.

"Thank you, Kevin," said Hedwig. "Ten Rand is a lot of money to people who have nothing, and she can save her son from a lifetime of misery now."

I was still in shock. My life had just turned full circle in front of my eyes and I didn't know whether to laugh or cry at the magic that was taking place around me on this misty track, thousands of miles from home.

I looked at my leg again and rubbed the long scar which ran down my knee. I had spent nearly the first six months of my life in hospital as a child. I had developed an infection in my knee at birth and nearly lost my leg, which doctors at first thought they could not save.

Yet a doctor, a stranger who I would never meet, who I would never know, had saved my leg after undertaking a long surgery on it thirty-five years ago.

A chill ran through me as I realised I had just helped save the leg of a child who would never know me either. And all it had taken was 80p and some incredible timing!

I sat quietly as we drove back to our next destination and my goose bumps had barely stopped tingling when Hedwig spoke.

"We are going to see a headmaster at another school now. He is a good man who helps many children and a charity has started running feeding schemes there now, following on from your project, Kevin."

"Wow!! That's fantastic news," I said. "How many children are being fed?" "The charity is working in another four schools, now. Thousands of children are receiving proper school meals because of this, but we do not know how long the charity will keep the schemes running for."

It had been my greatest hope that big charities would follow my example and run food to school projects here. I knew some Americans had visited at one time, and others from England too – and I had hoped someone with wealth would copy my simple scheme to feed children and help them go to school.

And at long last it was happening: an extra four thousand children a day were being fed now!

As my happiness peaked I looked at Sister with purpose and asked a question I soon wished I hadn't. "How many more schools are in Nkandla that don't receive any food yet?" She thought for a second. "More than a hundred, I think," she replied. My brief moment of delight deserted me as familiar feelings of despair were evoked once more.

I had fed over a quarter of a million school meals to the hungry children of Phalane Primary School myself by now, and had seemingly set wheels in motion which had led to many more children being fed each day – yet it was the thought of the tens of thousands of children who weren't being fed that concerned me.

Sister must have noticed my change in demeanour. "Kevin, you can't help them all. Keep the feeding scheme at Phalane running, and God will let it grow if it is his wish."

I'd almost forgotten. I had lost my part-time job before leaving home. It had sustained the project for so long now, and my savings had all but dried up. I didn't know how I was going to continue feeding the children at Phalane, let alone help anyone else.

One joy can scatter one hundred sorrows

Fighting Philosophy

The afternoon was to be as incredible as the morning as more mysterious coincidences and chance meetings led us to people who desperately needed our help.

To find someone on the road in need of a lift, to feed a hungry child wandering aimlessly down a dirt track, to lift the spirits of someone dying, or to smile and laugh with a child in desperate need of love. Each small act of humanity felt more profound than feeding thousands, and each event transpired in front of me as if at the desire of a higher will.

It was early evening by the time we arrived back at the convent and it had been a mind-blowing day. "We will be able to get something to eat shortly," said Sister, smiling as ever. "I'm going back to the guest house to wash up and relax a little first before I join you," I said.

It was still warm and bright and I slowly walked back to the guest house exhausted, thinking about all that had happened during the day.

I had felt powers at play which I couldn't explain, yet still struggled with the notion that a God was at work in this dreadful place.

If there really was an omnipotent force flowing through this universe, then where was it, why wasn't it down here sorting out the maddening manmade problems of the world?

I had experienced first-hand how little it took to make big changes over the last few years – even over the last few days, and the last few hours.

Maybe it was to do with free will. Free will didn't seem that *free* at the moment. It came at a high price. One man's free will seemed to come at the cost of another's.

I walked into the guest house and fell on the bed. I'd brought a newspaper with me from England, and picked it up for some light relief. But there was none to be found.

It was full of stories of crime, of tragedy, injustice and stupidity.

Stories of war in Iraq and Afghanistan filled the pages with tales of death and terror, intermingled sporadically with tips on how to lose weight and trivial celebrity gossip.

One article speculated the war in Iraq would cost the US $2 trillion by the time it was over, an incredible sum that could probably feed every child on the planet, instead of orphaning more.

"God, what's going on?" I sighed to myself as I got up briefly, before slumping down into a seat.

But there was no time for a midlife crisis here. The struggle to survive until tomorrow was a daily battle for most. I stared at the floor in contemplation, pondering my own mortality and my life's purpose. As I looked down, I saw a small ant scurry around aimlessly. "I know how you feel," I laughed as I watched on. It was a tiny creature compared to me; minute in fact. And although my foot was right next to it, it had absolutely no idea I was there watching its every move.

It had no idea who I was, or what I knew, or of the bigger universe around it. It could never experience life or the world in the way I could. It wasn't even conscious of thought. It just existed and experienced life in its own unique way – acting simply on instinct and compulsion.

I kept watching it with increasing intrigue. Was this like the nature of God compared to mankind? Were the gods that close to us, yet that almighty that we could not see them or recognise their presence – even if they were standing right next to us, like I was to the ant? Were we scurrying around desperately trying to find our way too, yet that out of phase with reality that we simply could not comprehend the nature of existence, just like the tiny ant could never comprehend me!

There was a knock on the door and I looked up. "Kevin," said Hedwig. "Are you coming for something to eat?"

"Yes," I shouted. "I'll be there in a minute."

I stood up, carefully avoiding the ant which had grown greatly in my appreciation, whilst looking around the room in amusement, in case a giant entity was standing next to me too.

I was hungry now – but more than that, I needed a beer. Quickly.

Those who question nothing, learn nothing

One Thousand to One

I woke in the morning with a headache. Not from the heavy conversations of spiritual philosophy with the nuns, but from one too many beers which had accompanied them.

It was my final day of three here, and later I would have to endure the long journey back home.

But before then, Sister had promised to take me to Phalane school to meet the headmaster and see the children I fed.

I went to breakfast but ate nothing, as I nursed a cup of tea to help shift my headache. Hedwig had arranged to meet me outside at 10am and I was looking forward to going to the school, as well as meeting one of the traders from whom I bought the fruits.

As I reached the car I saw Hedwig, who by now knew the routine well. "Would you like to go to town first to pick up some provisions for the drive out?" "Yes, please," I said, not knowing how many hungry children we would feed before the day's end.

After driving into town and emptying a bemused trader's stall of their produce, we headed out to Phalane. "The roads look a little better now than I remember on my previous trips, and there seem to be more building projects being undertaken," I said to her.

"Yes," replied Hedwig. "The roads have improved greatly and if the work continues in some areas, it will cut the travel time in and out of Nkandla and we will be able to take new routes safely."

"That's good," I said. "So things are improving here now." Sister looked at me sadly. "Only a little - people are still dying before their time and there is nothing we can do."

"Hasn't the Government extended the AIDS drugs trials yet?" I asked agitated by the indifference. "A charity is working here now," said Hedwig with a glimmer of hope. "They have put about 250 people on anti-retro viral drugs and are running the other school feeding schemes I told you about – but it isn't enough."

"I know," I sighed. "What about Lindiwe - is she receiving any treatment yet?" "No, her white blood cell count is still too high, but she is well. Would you like to see her after visiting Phalane?"

"Yes," I said, "I would."

It was about a twenty-minute drive to Phalane Primary School from the convent, but we stopped off at a few poor homesteads as we drove, passing out food parcels and fruit as we travelled.

Before long we reached Phalane and pulled up in a dusty cloud of smoke. I was to meet the trader here also, but she was late. When she finally arrived, she apologised profusely as I greeted her with a warm smile. She was a young mother, well-dressed and the proud owner of a truck - a rare asset for one her age. I knew she had benefited greatly from the contract to supply the school with fruit and I delighted in the knowledge that she was spreading this wealth as she spent her profit amongst other traders, expanding the fragile economy further.

When you put money in an area like Nkandla it stays there and gets spent over and over again. People are too poor to save money, and rarely have the opportunity to travel to spend it outside of the local community. Instead, it changes hands again and again, as one person's purchase becomes another person's sale.

Money I had spent eighteen months ago was still swirling around here somewhere, helping someone, and I laughed to myself at this remarkable side effect, which I had never planned.

"Tell her it's no problem," I said to Hedwig as we met, and the nervous woman calmed a little as Hedwig translated. It's funny how different people see you. To this young lady I must have seemed like a financial giant of great wealth and power. Yet back home I was just a normal bloke struggling to make a living like everyone else. Indeed, the most expensive thing I owned was a second-hand car worth less than £2,000, which was in desperate need of a service if truth be known!

It was break time at the school and as she unloaded the day's fruit, I looked around in amazement. It was the first time I had seen how many children I was actually feeding each day. I knew I fed 886 children – but that had just been a number up until now. But today I saw a sea of happy faces, each anxiously awaiting the fruit, and I suddenly realised what good the schemes were doing.

"Kevin," said Hedwig, waking me from my thoughts, "let's find Mr.

Mbatha in the main building over there."

"Okay," I said, as I followed her, feeling a little overwhelmed by the project I had set up.

We entered the office and I was immediately greeted by Mr. Mbatha and his deputy head whom I had met on my previous trip. "Banana Man" they said, shaking my hand as if I were a hero, "welcome, welcome."

Hedwig was laughing at my obvious discomfort. I don't really know what she thought of me, other than I was a good man at heart. But I think she was finally starting to realise that I was simply an ordinary person trying to do the right thing, and not the hero some here wrongly held me as.

Hedwig left the room so Mr. Mbatha could speak with me alone. "Thank you so much for helping our children," he said, holding himself professionally as I stood there unshaven in a dirty t-shirt and shorts. "That's OK," I said, still feeling uncomfortable at my apparent fame. "It has made such a difference to us here," he continued. "We will build a statue of you one day." I cringed with embarrassment, trying desperately not to turn red. "No it's OK, really. I think you can find something better to do with the money first."

I looked outside at the cramped conditions. "You could do with a large marquee tent to teach some of the children in, I think," I said, trying to smile off his previous comments. He misunderstood. "You will do that for us?" he asked excitedly. "Err, maybe…I'll try and bring you one on my next visit," I said, trying to backtrack quickly.

His eyes widened with delight. "Thank you, thank you," he said. He shook my hand again and asked me the question I had been dreading most, "You will keep feeding the children?"

I looked at him pensively, knowing I had just lost my job which had been financing the scheme. "You keep looking after the children and teaching them, and I'll keep feeding them," I said as my handshake sealed my promise.

"Please, you must tour the school and meet all the children and staff," said Mr. Mbatha as he led me from his office. "I will find the deputy head and she will escort you."

I walked outside and let out a deep breath as I rubbed my forehead in worry and I glanced at the floor. A nest of ants was busily working, and I remembered the ant in my room which had provoked my philosophical insight, and started laughing with a slight madness. The fates wanted me to keep feeding the children here, and who was I to argue with them – even if I didn't know how I could.

Hedwig rejoined me with the deputy head and we were given a grand tour of the school. "I think I owe Mr. Mbatha a marquee," I whispered to Hedwig as she looked at me, puzzled. As we walked we were told that because of the feeding schemes, the number of children in Phalane had now swelled to over a thousand children, as more and more migrated to the school, just to receive a little fruit!

We continued through the school and I was introduced to sixteen teachers, who each greeted me warmly as 'Banana Man' as they shook my hand or hugged me.

I felt like a fish out of water, a reluctant hero to a desperate people. I was over my head and at the end of my ability to help them any further, but I couldn't bring myself to tell them…

We left the school and I smiled philosophically to Sister. "I'd better put a lottery ticket on when I get home," I said with half a smile. She didn't understand what I meant but smiled back regardless.

If the fates existed, they seemed to torment and challenge, and I knew my pound bet would be better spent here any day, than on a ticket of chance; but then destiny had many surprises install for me yet, unbeknown to me.

They that never climbed, never fell

For the Love of Lindiwe

My trip was rapidly coming to an end, but there was just enough time to visit the Lindiwe homestead before we headed back to the convent for my departure.

I sat in contemplation as we drove, and Hedwig left me to my thoughts. I had wanted to be a magic wand for her and end her hellish world with the swish of a wrist. But I hadn't been able to do this in nearly two years.

Why I even thought I could make changes here was beyond me; in fact I had never once thought that I could – I had just constantly felt I *should*, and that feeling never left me, not day or night.

Sometimes the answers seemed so simple. They were almost within my grasp, so clear and pure; but for some reason they were always just out of reach, and this brought great frustration as a world of petty distractions stopped me from my task. I knew the simplest way to help Sister now was to fill her with the hope that I was trying hard to change her plight and that of her people.

Confirming the continuation of the scheme at Phalane had done just that, but I didn't know what the future held for either of us.

All I knew was that we were going to visit Lindiwe next and it was a miracle in itself that she was still alive. But then she had angels like Hedwig and the other Sisters willing her to live.

We slowly climbed the familiar mountain road towards Lindiwe's home and stopped the car just short of the top. "She has a fantastic view to wake up to each morning," I said to Hedwig as I looked out at the beauty of the surrounding landscape.

We took the last food we had with us and walked the steep track down to her home. The sisters had received some donations from Catholics in America, and used this money to help build Lindiwe a brick house, which was a massive jump in living conditions for her and her family.

"Is Lindiwe here?" I asked Hedwig, looking around at the children playing. Hedwig called out and an elderly lady came from a hut and spoke with us. "This is Lindiwe's mother," said Hedwig. "Lindiwe has gone to town and won't be back for a few hours, but we can leave the food here for her and the children."

I had intended to give Lindiwe the last of the money I had and felt disappointed to have missed her. But we played with the children for a while and gave them some fruit and sweets before leaving.

As we left I handed the old lady the last of my money, which quickly disappeared into her pocket as she thanked me with a smile that said a thousand words. Hedwig had seen me and was laughing. "It was for Lindiwe and the children," I said. "Do you think the old granny will give it to her when she comes home?"

"Not a chance," laughed Hedwig, and I smiled as we headed back to the convent, knowing the money would go to great use anyway.

I have not failed.
I've just found 10,000 ways that won't work.
Thomas Edison

Zulu Time

As we arrived at the convent the Sisters were preparing for my departure, and had made me some food, which I ate only out of courtesy for their efforts.

Sister Hedwig left me for a while, and returned a short time later with a letter and gift for Joanne and my children. "What is this?" I enquired.

"I know how difficult it is for your family when you leave them to come here and help people they do not know," said Hedwig. "It must put a lot of stress on them and this letter is to thank them from me."

I nodded in appreciation and put the items in my now empty suitcase, before walking outside with Hedwig, where each of the Sisters blessed me with a loving hug.

"We will see you again, I think, Kevin," said Sister Michaelis, smiling as she hugged me, and I knew she had seen into my heart long ago.

I nodded knowingly to her, and climbed into the car where I was met by a smiling face. I was to be driven back to the different world of Durban by a local Zulu called Norman who worked for the nuns as a driver. As Norman started the car, I bade my friends a final farewell and waved goodbye as we pulled away.

Norman was a typical Zulu, happy and friendly despite his poor position in life.

We talked for most of the journey back to Durban, and the parallels between our lives were uncanny.

As well as these parallels though, there were some stark differences too. Norman told me about some of the Zulu traditions that are still held today, and how he had met his wife to be a long time ago.

The price of a Zulu marriage was far higher than true love, and he was forced to pay a fifteen-cow dowry to his father-in-law before he could wed the woman of his heart.

Each cow cost hundreds of pounds – huge sums of money to the average Zulu, even if they were lucky enough to be one of the few in paid employment like Norman. He had been paying one cow at a time for many years now, but still had seven cows to pay before he could marry the girl of his dreams!

He was thirty five like me, but still faced a seven-year wait to wed because of his enormous dowry debt!

"Wow, that's true love," I said in amazement as he told me his story. "Most people in Britain have married and divorced by the time you will have saved up to marry your wife."

Norman laughed, but his plight was harsh in a land already ravaged by poverty and disease. Life expectancy was low here and he would be in his forties before he could wed.

"Why don't you ask for a discount?" I joked. "Tell your father-in-law his daughter was worth fifteen cows when you met her eight years ago, but by the time she is in her forties you will both have lost so much time together – that it's not worth the same amount anymore."

Norman wasn't used to my Liverpudlian sense of humour, but was wetting himself laughing as we joked, and I regularly had to point his attention back to the road. "Yes, I will," he said. "Then I will run for my life!" "Who from, the wife or the father-in-law?" I asked as tears poured down his face. "Both!" he exclaimed.

We kept laughing and joking as we drove and slowly, surely, sadly, the scenery changed from abject poverty to opulent wealth. The battered trucks and carts turned to Mercedes and 4 x 4s; large houses appeared in the place of shacks, shops materialised, large modern schools and people too. There's a grey point which you pass where this transformation begins, and it's a bizarre sight to witness with open eyes.

The tiring drive took little less than four hours in total, and as we pulled into Durban's heaving airport, I knew I had made another unlikely friend in Norman.

He had brought me back to civilisation safely, but faced a long drive home and it would be dark and dangerous by the time he arrived back in Nkandla. I had saved a little cash to pay for petrol, but handed it to Norman and told him to save it towards his next cow. "And don't forget to ask for a discount!" I yelled as he drove away, happy and grateful for his large tip.

I hated the painful return to society and the wealth of the west, but walked into the airport feeling less stressed than on previous homecomings.

The same scenes of unawareness surrounded me as I walked past people lost to life and the horrors only a few hundred miles away. I entered the same restaurant I had on my last journey, but felt different now, almost happy. My travels were enriching me and making me appreciate each day of life as a precious gift.

Each day held wonder and awe for me now, and nothing could take this away.

I had lost weight, as usual, and needed to eat, so sat down and ordered a meal, which I ate with an appreciation I had not felt before. As I did, I recalled the incredible moments of the last few days and they uplifted my spirits to new heights. I giggled childishly as I realised I would never know the ripple effects of my actions, or the results of the wheels I had set in motion.

Our actions today ripple long into the future, I realised as I ate hungrily.

Then I saw in my mind the people I had given cash to, knowing this money would continue to spread magic through their lives and those of others, long after their faces had faded from my memory.

I finished my meal and knew I needed to call Joanne and let her know I was safe. She would be going out of her mind by now again. As I walked down the stairs to buy a phone card, I heard the loud roar of a plane as it took to the sky.

I was exhausted but still faced three uncomfortable flights before I would be home.

I really hated flying…

What is right is often forgotten by what is convenient
Bodie Thoene

New Purpose, Old Madness

I arrived home later the next day to a tearful welcome from Joanne, Rebecca and James. They didn't understand why I had left them again and they hadn't liked it.

We had sacrificed a family holiday together and I knew this precious time was lost forever. Maybe one day they would understand why I had had to go back to Africa, and forgive me.

I had only been back home a few days when Trevor rang me to apologise and ask me to go back and work for him on better terms. I agreed, but knew I needed more from life, and had to do something different if I was to truly help the children I had left behind in Nkandla.

Nevertheless, I returned to the job and went back working long hours which allowed me to pay for the fruit to feed the children of Phalane, which had now swelled in numbers to more than a thousand.

Joanne was still struggling to cope with the changing processes I was going through, and she had hoped with each trip I would clear my system and return to normality. But reality itself had changed for me. I could no more stop the transformation I was going through than a caterpillar could stop turning into a butterfly as it found its wings to fly.

With the end of each trip a new journey started; this came with familiar family frustrations, as I struggled to find a new way forward.

I still needed to raise £40,000 to secure and expand my scheme and feed and educate more children.

It was soon late December and Christmas was coming quickly. I had been promising Joanne I would take her Christmas shopping for ages, and the day had finally arrived. I'd taken half a day off work and wanted some lunch before braving the crushing Christmas crowds of town.

As I sipped my soup, I sat watching TV racking my brains how I could raise more money, when a news report came on talking of Britain's Trident replacement ambitions. The UK owned forty-eight nuclear weapons, each with the awesome power to kill a million people within seconds of their detonation.

Now politicians were trying to replace these ageing weapons with some brand new ones. The cost of this was set at a staggering £76 billion, including annual maintenance costs over the next thirty years and could have fed **1.9 trillion** meals to the hungry.

Whilst mankind let around 30,000 children die of hunger and poverty every day, we were planning for war thirty years into the future, and the world looked doomed never to be at peace.

"Why is all this money available for weapons, when we can't find money to feed kids," I grumbled to myself as Joanne walked into the room. "I don't know," she said, impatiently waiting for me to finish my soup so we could go shopping.

"No wonder this world is in such a state when so many politicians are disconnected with the plight of ordinary people".

I knew it wasn't just me that felt this way. Trust in politicians was rapidly crumbling. This month Tony Blair had just become the first ever British prime minister to be questioned by police in the course of an investigation. This particular investigation was in relation to bribery and corruptions allegations linked to the 'cash for honours' scandal. Donations seemed to have been traded for peerages and the scandal had been rumbling on for most of the year. Mr Blair was one in a long line of labour party members, ministers, and Lords to be questioned or arrested over the matter…and the other main political parties seemed very quiet on the subject, given its seriousness.

"Look, can we go shopping and put the world to rights later?" Joanne asked as she put her coat on.

I felt isolated again, like I had so often over the last two years. Was there nothing I could do to save the Zulu?

I knew I had to do more. I had to keep trying.

"Come on!" shouted Joanne, and I got my coat and left to go Christmas shopping.

None so blind as those who will not see

Crimes Against Humanity

All too soon Christmas came, and I enjoyed the rest and relaxation with my family.

Since starting the Phalane feeding scheme I knew I had fed nearly three hundred thousand school meals of fresh fruit to the hungry children there. When term started again next year, I would feed a thousand more meals a day – yet I knew tens of thousands more children were left to go hungry.

I was determined to do more, but really at a loss what to do next. I'd tried fundraising and to obtain grants last year, only to chase my tail without success.

On top of this I'd written to millionaires, billionaires and businesses, telling them of my efforts and the dreadful plight of the Zulus. Most didn't reply, and those that did sent sympathetic letters, but nothing more.

I often pondered why fate had drawn *me* to Nkandla, instead of people with great wealth or power, when I was so helpless to save the children. The only real quality I had was a stubborn will which wouldn't allow me to give up.

As New Years Eve came I accepted that I had gone bananas long ago – but held out hope that I wasn't quite crazy just yet. I was having a lazy day as I sat watching the morning news, as it revealed that Saddam Hussein had been executed for crimes against humanity.

Britain had joined the war against Iraq in 2003. At least a million ordinary people had marched on London in protest - the UK's largest ever demonstration - yet they were still ignored by the politicians in power, and we started a disastrous war that was ripping the country apart.

"No wonder this world is so screwed up," I said to Joanne as she walked into the room. "They have just killed Saddam Hussein for crimes against humanity."

"Didn't he deserve to die?" said Joanne "He was a dictator who killed thousands of his own people."

"Maybe," I said, "But what about the other crimes against humanity?"

I knew that millions of native South Africans had been left to die unnecessarily from poverty as a pandemic had struck them so cruelly. It was estimated by 2010 as many as twenty percent of all children in South Africa would be AIDS orphans, ironically the same year as FIFA would hold the world cup there. And I feared in twenty or thirty years' time, the indigenous Zulus of Nkandla could well be extinct because of a neglect that was nothing short of genocide in my mind.

But it wasn't just South Africa. My travels had opened my eyes, and I looked around the world in great pain, as I realised how powerful governments and business had let down the lost children of the world, whilst pursuing personal self interest and wealth.

Statistics showed that across the globe as many as one billion children lived in poverty: 640 million lived without adequate shelter, 400 million had no access to safe water, 270 million had no access to health services. The figures were staggering.

Unforgivably, eleven million frightened children were still dying of hunger and poverty each year and most would die quietly, out of the scrutiny and conscience of the 'civilised' world.

Yet each and every one of these children has as much right to exist as we do – and to live in peace and hope and happiness.

I had left home two years ago to save a dying child, only to become an accidental father to a thousand more. Now I looked around the world and saw hundreds of millions of desperate children who needed help.

Crimes against humanity were happening every day all over the world. And the evil veil of illusion that shrouded them needed to be lifted.

When I give food to the poor, they call me a saint.
When I ask why the poor have no food,
they call me a communist.
Dom Helda Camara

New Year, New Hope

As 2006 came to a close, I brought in the New Year with my family, attending a party at my local karate club. I used to look at the New Year as an opportunity to make resolutions, and a chance for change and self-improvement; but had learnt long ago I must do this daily.

I didn't know what the year ahead held for me - who does? But as it began I was feeding a thousand children a day, single handedly, and feeling burnt out, at my wit's end, and shamefully close to giving up...

I needed something to change, and I needed it to change fast.

A few days later I quit my part-time job in order to take control of my destiny once more and to try and live my dreams.

But then my dreams hadn't always gone to plan in the past. A few years earlier I had created a unique diary and patented it. It had the potential of turning the diary industry on its head, and at first they had shown great interest in my concept. In those days I thought I'd make my fortune through licensing off my idea worldwide, but ultimately the manufacturers did not produce them. Despite this, I knew my diary design was a real winner, so I produced a sample batch myself, only to struggle to sell them.

I'd put my heart and soul into creating the diaries back then, and with a rejuvenated zest, spent January trying to earn some extra cash by selling the ones I had left from stock, with little success.

Strange coincidences were still happening to me regularly though, and a chance encounter, early February, led me to attend a business networking meeting in London.

At first I thought about promoting my diary concept at the meeting, but as I travelled to London my mind was consumed with the plight of the children - and how on earth I was going to keep the feeding schemes going...

I looked out of the train window as the scenery sped by, and the choice became simple - I would have to talk of Africa when I arrived at the meeting.

It was Monday morning, and I needed strong coffee to calm my nerves when I arrived, as I felt uncomfortable at having to stand up and talk. I spoke publicly for the first time about what had happened to me over the last two years and as people listened intently, I had no idea what the week ahead was to bring.

By Tuesday, one of the well connected businessmen in the room had told many of his contacts about my efforts, and throughout the day I was inundated with emails offering support and useful contacts.

By Wednesday I had been asked to write a book about my adventures to help raise awareness for the children, and received offers of many valuable services worth thousands of pounds.

By Thursday I had spoken with people the length and breadth of the UK, and from every corner of the globe - including France, Brussels,

Japan, Singapore, America and New Zealand. These people were kindly offering help and advice, words of support, free services, and donations – but more than that, friendship.

By Friday I had been invited to speak on the radio in London, as well as receiving sponsorship to feed thousands more children, more offers of help, and more kind words of support.

In the coming months I would be featured in various magazines and local newspapers, as well as being asked to talk at events as far afield as London, Manchester, Holland and Germany.

Later, I would speak on Canadian and South African radio to audiences of hundreds of thousands.

Having felt so isolated over the last two years, my life was turning on its head again, as people began to here my story and join in my quest to save the forgotten children of Zululand.

But in truth my journey was only just beginning…

Example is not the main thing in influencing others
It's the only thing
Albert Schweitzer

Just One Child

At this time I didn't run a charity, and had pretty much done everything on my own – but it was becoming clear I needed a vehicle to fundraise through. At first I contacted the documentary makers to see if I could fundraise through the trust they had set up to help the children in Nkandla, but they were difficult to pin down, and often away in other countries on filming assignments, and seemed to have moved on. Then, a charity called Just One Child, which helped orphaned children in South Africa, heard of my work and offered to act as an umbrella for my feeding schemes.

By early May things were going well and I was running up and down the country, giving speeches here, there and everywhere. This allowed me to highlight the plight of Zululand's forgotten AIDS orphans, as well as raising some much needed cash to sustain the feeding schemes.

At each event I spoke passionately on behalf of the children, reliving the emotional rollercoaster ride which had been my life for the last two years. As I told my stories I seemed to move people greatly, yet each time I spoke, deep emotions stirred within me, and I soon felt out of sync with everyone in the room, wishing I was back in Africa helping the children instead of giving talks to groups of strangers.

It was a bizarre period of time for me. Not least because I was a private person, yet I kept finding myself the centre of attention in crowded rooms. Hearty handshakes from business people with a pat on the back and a "well done to you". Warm smiles and hugs, with words of adulation from people I'd never met.

Yet while I was being showered in praise, children were still left to a terrible fate, and despite meeting people of power, I just never seemed able to build enough momentum or funding to achieve my goals. I pushed on anyway, in the belief that one day, someone would hear my words and respond in the profound way needed to save the children.

I'd just returned from a talk in Surrey, when a major breakthrough came and I was contacted by a national tabloid who had heard of my story. The excited journalist wanted to write an article on my work, indeed on my whole family and the impact it had had on our lives. They interviewed both Joanne and me for hours over the phone, and the next day a photographer from London travelled to see us and took pictures; soon after this, the journalist sent us a draft copy of the article they would be publishing that Sunday.

The whole affair was a bit of a whirlwind for us, and I wasn't quite sure that I wanted to be featured in the national press as 'Banana Man' holding a five foot blow-up banana and bunches of fruit! Nevertheless, the article had the potential of making people aware of the plight of the Zulus, and the paper had promised to make a large donation to my work too.

"Wow Kevin, this could create a lot of publicity for the children," Joanne said excitedly. "I know" I said, hopeful that this was the turning point which was desperately needed.

A few days later and the plight of another child filled the papers. The story travelled the world like wildfire. The story of just one child - Madeleine McCann.

News of Madeleine's disappearance shocked the country, and hit the headlines only days before the story of South Africa's AIDS orphans was due to be published.

As Madeleine's story broke, all other news became displaced, and the national newspaper which was to feature the plight of the Zulu children, dropped my story.

Madeleine was only three when she had been abducted whilst on holiday in Portugal with her family.

I think most parents had lost sight of their children for a moment at one time or another and it's a truly sickening feeling when it happens. When Rebecca was three we'd lost her for a few minutes in a shopping complex in Liverpool. At that age she would run around non-stop, and she'd broken away from us as we were looking in a shop window. As we saw her disappear through a sea of legs, we were panic-stricken. She could move really quickly for her size, and in a flash she was gone. We had security looking for her as we ran around the mall shouting her name in panic. In the few terrifying minutes it took to find her, frightful thoughts ran through our minds, and by the time we found her sitting happily in a 20p coin-slot ride, I didn't know whether to kiss her or kill her!

It was every parent's worst nightmare to have their child abducted, and Madeleine's plight dominated the headlines daily as the nation's interest grew in the case like no other before it.

Like everyone else, we took a great interest in the case, hoping that the search for Madeleine would find her safe and well quickly, but it wasn't to be.

By early August I was preparing to travel to Holland to teach at the country's largest martial arts festival for charity. On the day of travel I entered the airport and bought a newspaper to read during the short flight to Amsterdam.

Attention for the whereabouts of Madeleine had continued month after month and sightings were reported in different countries from time to time.

Today the newspapers headline read that Madeleine had been spotted by a child therapist who claimed that she was "100% sure" she had seen her at a restaurant in a Belgian town near the Dutch border, only days earlier.

I found it bizarre that I would be in Holland as the search for Madeleine suddenly switched its focus there, and I soon found myself thinking back to my first journey to find Sne. In fact it was that initial trip to Africa which was the reason I was travelling to Holland this very day to fundraise. I remembered how Madeleine's abduction had stopped the story of the Zulu's being run in the press, and how the world would be a better place if humanity responded to the plight of all children in need.

Luckily, it was only a short flight to Amsterdam and it wasn't long before I was in the air. As we rose through the clouds I looked out of the window and started to think of the amazing things humankind were capable of; what they had achieved and where we were heading.

After all, here I was, sitting strapped to a seat inside hundreds of tonnes of metal with massive engines, travelling at breathtaking speed through the air with the grace of a bird!

As the plane continued to climb I looked down as the ground became smaller and smaller, and realised that I lived in incredible times. Even our most basic day was full of wonder. Today, I could do anything. I could eat foods from the four corners of the world, foods that even kings of old would never have tasted. I had access to knowledge that time's greatest scientists struggled to fathom, and I utilised technology that history's most ingenious inventors couldn't have dreamt of. I could see a world that our forefathers never knew existed, and go places where history's greatest explorers had never trod.

Mankind had reached to the stars and grasped them with both hands. We had travelled to the moon, sent spacecraft to Mars, created language, art, music and culture. We had explored the deepest oceans and even delved into the genetic make up of life itself! We seemed capable of achieving anything our imagination could conceive; yet the simplest things still seemed to elude us. With all our powers, with all our will, we still couldn't find one little girl, so cruelly taken from her parents.

I was soon in Holland and the rest of the weekend passed quickly and was pleasant, if tiring. I met some old friends there, and made some news ones, but as I returned to the UK, I walked straight back into life's daily, trivial, problems.

Despite my initial successes, I was pretty hopeless when it came to fundraising - and I was a long way from achieving my target of feeding more children.

But if I was nothing else, I was a fighter, and I held out hope.

A Wrong to put Right

So much had happened to me since my first trip to Africa, and as November approached, I was looking forward to returning to Nkandla.

But before I did, there was something I desperately wanted to do for Hedwig – and I had been putting it off for too long.

Her brother had died over a year ago, yet I knew she was still plagued by her belief that he had gone to 'hell' as a non-practising Catholic. This was dreadful to my mind, and it wasn't the message I thought Catholicism was preaching in the UK anyway, so reluctantly decided to visit a local Catholic church, and ask the priest for clarification.

I felt uncomfortable with this unwanted duty; after all who was I to ask this question and what was I going to say anyway? "Hi Father, I don't believe in Catholicism, but I need to ask a question about your beliefs to help a nun in Africa…can tell me if you think people go to hell just because they're not Catholics!"

Crumbs, I'd probably get thrown out of the chapel and arrested for disturbing the peace, or worse, dragged to confession or preached to for hours!

"Why me?" I thought to myself as I drove reluctantly towards the church. I arrived all too soon, and as I walked up the path, I just wanted to turn around and run. "Maybe I should go and put a shirt and tie on" I thought, as I rang the doorbell, trying to find any excuse to leave whilst I still had the chance.

The bell rang out loudly, and a few seconds later a little old lady struggled to open the large wooden door, which creaked stubbornly under the strain. As she came into sight, she caught my eye before looking me up and down awkwardly. "Yes, what is it you want?" she asked bluntly, as she stared at me blankly.

"Is the priest here, I need to talk to him", I said softly. "Who, Father Ned? He's having his lunch, can I pass him a message?"

"Oh, erm - no" I said uncomfortably. "It's…well…it's a private matter, I'll come back another time."

The lady looked at me again, and must have sensed I had no intention of returning if I left now. "No, please come in – I'll find Father for you if you wait in here."

I entered the building and I was escorted to a small sitting room to wait. I don't know what it is about churches, but for me they're like hospitals, and have a certain feel and smell about them, which puts you on edge, rather than at ease. The room was small, old fashioned and simply furnished with a table and a few chairs. I sat up stiffly, surveying the room's various religious pictures and symbols which adorned the walls, and I began to hope that Father Ned was still eating and too busy to see me.

I still didn't have a clue what I was going to say to him anyway. I'd brought some photographs and some news clippings to help me break the ice, and got them out of my backpack as I thought I better try and explain some of the background before I popped him the big question.

The few minutes wait seemed to last an age, and as I watched each second slowly tick by on the clock, I wanted to get up and sneak out unnoticed. But I knew I had to stay. I had to stay for Hedwig.

Father Ned eventually entered the room. I'd been told by Joanne that his real name was 'Father Ted' but that he had changed it to Ned because of the link to the popular comedy series on TV, which poked fun at the Catholic Church. Why I had to think of this just as he walked in the room I don't know. But the second I saw him I had to stop myself from laughing.

"Hello, I'm Father Ned" said a soft Irish voice as pictures of 'Father Ted and Dougal' from the TV comedy flashed through my mind. I put my hand to my mouth and coughed to stifle my laugh. "How can I help you?" he continued.

The humour of the moment helped relax me a little and I quickly composed myself. "It's a long story, Father", I said. "They always are," he replied with a faint smile. "It's usually best to start from the beginning."

Father was right, so I spent the next ten minutes telling him of the events of the last few years which had led me to Africa, and which had now brought me to him in need of his advice. As I finished, I explained that the Sisters believed all non-Catholics were doomed to an eternity in hell – and that this belief brought much torment to Sister Hedwig, who had lost her parents and brother to AIDS.

Father Ned seemed almost angry that such things were still being taught. "No, it is not our belief that people go to hell, simply because they aren't Catholic," he said. "I know this used to be taught a long time ago in certain parts of the world, but I'm surprised that such things are still being taught."

I looked at Father anxiously. "I'm returning to Zululand soon – will you write me a letter to confirm this to Sister Hedwig, to put her mind at ease?" "It's difficult," he said tentatively as he gazed at me in thought. "I don't want to confuse someone who has been brought to find God with these strong views." I understood completely. I had wanted to tell Sister that her brother hadn't gone to hell a thousand times, but each time I tried, I couldn't find the words, and feared I would cause her more pain if I expressed my opinions.

Father Ned could sense my disappointment. "Kevin, let me read some of your literature, then I will write a letter for Sister."

"Thank you, Father," I said in delight, knowing that a carefully worded letter from a priest would bring great comfort to Hedwig.

I left the church and was glad when I arrived back home after my ordeal. Father had said he would call me after looking at my website and reading more about my work, and true to his word, a few days later I received a call from him.

"Kevin, I cannot believe what you have been doing for our Catholic family," he said excitedly. "I do it for the children, not the church," I said, feeling as uncomfortable as ever at the unwanted attention.

"We must help you in any way we can," he continued. "I want to get our whole community behind your work. You must come and speak to the congregation and tell them what you have done. They are very generous and we will hold a collection to support your work." "Thank you," I said, "I need all the support I can get at the moment."

"Kevin, I am attending a local school later today as part of my community work. I will speak to the children and tell them your story and ask the school to help you too." "Thank you," I said. "And the letter? I'm returning to Africa in a few weeks. Will you still write a letter for me to take to Sister Hedwig?"

"Yes, of course," said Father Ned. "We'll speak again before you go, and I will write you a letter to help better explain the position of the church."

As I got off the phone I felt a great relief, hoping Sister Hedwig's unnecessary torment would soon finally come to an end.

The Case of the Condoms

The next few weeks passed quickly and it wasn't long before I was returning to Africa. Despite the fact it was my fourth journey to Zululand, it was the first time I had had the luxury to plan for it.

Sister Hedwig had been in contact with me by email all year and she was excited by the news I was returning. She'd made arrangements to pick me up at Durban airport, and knew I always brought a suitcase packed with children's clothes and toys to support her work. But the tone of her emails had changed over the last few months, as she had been asked to leave the job she loved as a social worker helping children, in order to support the Sisters more in their work.

email from Africa.......

Dear Kevin...
....I am actually writing to tell you of some changes that have taken place since last week. I know you will not understand it because it is the way of life I have chosen. Recently I received a letter from the church in Germany telling me to move out of the hospital and give up my job in capacity as a Social Worker and to go and support Sister Ellen in her work...this has disturbed me so much to leave my work...

I had never understood the politics of the church, but had ignored them in the past when they had surfaced. I often forgot that the Sister's first mission was to God, not people, but could feel her heartbreak at having to leave her post, where she helped look after nearly a thousand needy children.

I knew at least she would still be working in the community as grass roots level, and having developed a network of contacts over the year, I was being asked if I needed anything to take with me on my pending journey.

I thought long and hard about what the people needed most, and I desperately wanted to stop the spread of AIDS, which continued to create more orphans daily. Food, clothes and toys were cheap enough to buy on the ground in South Africa, and besides I could only carry 20-kilos of baggage on the plane. Anti-retro viral drugs were too expensive, and I wasn't a doctor qualified to dispense them anyway, so this wasn't a good idea either.

I remembered from my previous trips that the nuns gave out condoms when they were able as a prevention measure, and I knew these were hard to come by in rural areas, and impossibly expensive to people who didn't have enough money for food or other basic necessities.

Condoms were light enough to carry in volume and would help save lives. So I put out an email to my contacts; Nuns need Condoms!

I'm not sure Father Ned would have particularly approved of my request, but then I was struggling to pin him down for the letter he had promised to write for me anyway. I made numerous calls to the church, but he was always out. On the day before I travelled, I made a desperate final attempt to secure a letter from him, but he had gone away for a few days, and the opportunity to ease Hedwig's burden was lost.

Sadness had been my companion these last years, but this was an unnecessary disappointment. Father Ned's promise of a letter to Hedwig had meant so much to me. But there was no time for self-pity today; I had to prepare for the journey ahead.

One of my friends had told me they had sourced a large donation of condoms a few weeks earlier, but on the day of travel they still hadn't arrived, so I filled my suitcase with children's clothes and toys instead.

I was flying later that evening and as midday approached the doorbell rang, and I opened the door to face a smirking courier.

"I've got ten kilo's of condoms here for a 'Banana Man' " he said. I looked at the enormous carton he was delivering, before looking back at him blankly. "Just don't ask," I said straight-faced, as I signed for the parcel, before shutting the door quickly, to the sound of his sniggers.

"Joanne!" I shouted. "The condoms have just arrived and we need to repack my suitcase quickly if I'm to take them."

Joanne was more relaxed with me travelling this time, but she didn't seem over impressed I was travelling with a suitcase full of condoms!

She opened up one of the boxes, then burst into laughter – "Kevin you can't take these, the packets have pictures of a naked woman on the front, you'll give the nuns a heart attack!"

I looked at one of the boxes and cringed. The condoms had been donated via the music television station MTV, and were obviously given out at out gigs and concerts to promote safe sex.

If the provocative naked lady on the front wasn't bad enough, the boxes were marked as "Limited Edition, Ultra Feeling Condoms, plus 1 Surprise!"

"Ooo – I've just found the surprise," said Joanne in fits of laughter, "it's a chocolate one." Then, as she delved deeper into the box, she found another surprise and creased up in hysterics. "Look what's in each pack," she said with tears running down her face.

MTV had kindly enclosed helpful pictures of the kama sutra in each packet of condoms, to help show users how to perform such acrobatically impressive sex acts as 'The Wheel'.

By now all I could do was laugh "Oh no – I can't take these to the nuns, I'll get thrown out!"

"Listen," said Joanne, "there are too many boxes to fit in your suitcase anyway, let's unpack them all and you can just take the loose condoms."

"We'll have to," I said, as we set about shelling box after box and putting thousands of loose condoms into my case. "I've helped you do some crazy things in the past, Kevin," Joanne said, looking at me, "but this really takes the biscuit."

"At least you don't have to walk through customs with them," I said, as Joanne gestured a security guard snapping a tight rubber glove to his hand. "Not on your life!" I cried, shaking my head in horror at the thought!

The hour was late, and soon after packing my case it was time for me to leave for Africa once more. James and Rebecca were both at school, so leaving wasn't as emotional as usual, thankfully.

We'd all been out for a meal the night before, and I think my family accepted my need to go to Zululand more now, than perhaps they had in the past. James had looked me in the eyes before he left for school in the morning and told me in a very serious voice, not to get shot. It was the only moment of doubt I had before I left - not because I feared being shot, but because my eight-year-old son feared I might.

This was small comfort to Joanne who was worried sick as she waved me off, and I knew deep down, her worst fear was that she would never see me again.

After an hour's drive, I arrived at Manchester airport, knowing I faced travelling through various security points here, as well as in Paris, Johannesburg and Durban – with a case packed full of loose condoms and very little else.

I waited in the long check-in queue for an age, worried about the contents of my case, and the questions which would arise as I tried to check it in.

Sadly, we still lived in an age of terror and only a few months ago two Iraqi doctors had tried to explode a flaming Jeep into Glasgow airports departure lounge - and I knew the thousands of tiny silver foiled packages which filled my case to the brim, were likely to cause a major panic when X-rayed by security!

As I stood in line I contemplated the ludicrous world we lived in. The government had long been threatening to bring in compulsory biometric data cards to improve airport security in their fight against terror. But the scheme was set to cost the UK tax payer a colossal £18 billion over ten years – enough to feed **450 billion** meals of fruit to hungry children! Luckily, most people didn't trust the government's motives – let alone their ability to hold their DNA safely. Only last month they'd lost my personal bank details along with those of 25 million other people - and I didn't need ministers to tell me they weren't fit for purpose.

Thankfully, ID cards had been Tony Blair's brainchild, and he'd been ousted from power earlier in the year by his own party. He had long lost his credibility with the British public and become an electoral liability to New Labour. Illegal wars, death and destruction, missing weapons of mass destruction and cash for honours scandals were to be his legacy now.

This had allowed Gordon Brown to wrestle his way to power, but he was faring no better, and soon faced the lowest rating of any prime minister since the 1950's, when Eden had colluded with France to go to war against Egypt so they could seize control of the Suez canal.

War and terror were nothing new, sadly…and the world seemed to be built on domination and Empire.

A camp voice broke me sharply from my thoughts. "Next, please." I looked towards the check-in desk to face the clerk who was taking great pleasure in flaunting the fact he was gay. "Can you pop your case up here for me, Sir?" "Sure," I said in a manly voice, now more nervous than ever to discuss its contents. "And where are you going to today?" he asked in feminine tones as he inspected my ticket… "Oooh Africa, that's nice."

"Yes, I'm visiting nuns," I said quickly, as he shot me an enquiring glance. "I'm taking supplies to them in my case," I continued, desperately struggling to explain myself. "It's full of thousands of condoms!" I blurted out, not knowing what else to say. He tipped his glasses to look me up and down for a moment. "They're needed to help stop the spread of AIDS," I said, as I felt myself shrink smaller and smaller. "Well…I think we need to put a note on your case then, Sir, to help it pass through customs safely," he said mischievously.

I continued waffling awkwardly, but I was just digging myself into a bigger hole each time I spoke. "I know it looks strange to carry this many condoms out of their packets, but I had to take them all out of the boxes because of the naked woman on the front of the box… and…the nuns…you see…". "Oh, it's OK, Sir, you don't need to explain yourself to me," he said as he passed back my ticket. "Besides, it sounds like you are going to have a fabulous time in Africa. It's just a shame I can't come with you."

By now I had turned crimson and I grabbed my ticket, put my head down in shame, and left as fast as my legs could carry me, without looking back.

How I ended up in these situations in life, I don't know. I had never planned to feed a thousand children a day, or do any of the crazy things which happened to me regularly now; they just seemed to take on a life of their own. All I knew was I needed a strong coffee, and some quiet time to regain my composure before the trip ahead.

A trip which was plain sailing - until I reached Johannesburg a day later...

Plain Sailing

The flights through to Johannesburg were as uncomfortable and tiring as always and I was looking forward to having my feet back on the ground at they came to an end.

As we started our descent, the seat belt sign came on and the captain spoke over the tannoy and gave us a brief weather report, mumbling something about the civil aviation authority, and thanking us for flying with Air France.

Air France always gave out their announcements in French first, then gave a short inaudible version in English, so I never took much notice.

Twenty minutes later and we had landed, and I needed to race to collect my luggage if I was going to make my connecting flight to Durban, so I quickly made my way through the terminal. "I wonder if my suitcase made it this far," I thought as I went through passport control – before stumbling into scenes of bedlam.

"What is happening here?", a voice from behind me said. I turned to see a large white South African woman who was obviously in a hurry too. "I don't know," I said in bemusement, "but it doesn't look good."

I went to find my luggage and pushed my way through the teeming crowds of angry commuters who filled every corner of the terminal. A large group of passengers had surrounded a lone figure, who was desperately trying to answer questions and pacify the mob, so I headed in her direction.

"Do you know what's happening?" I asked a young couple in front of me.

"We think an engine has fallen off a plane as it was taking off" they said, "and the civil aviation authority has grounded all flights for safety reasons."

"Only in Africa," exclaimed a well dressed businessman who had been listening in, trying to glean information.

Rumours abounded, but it soon became clear that my next airline, Nationwide, had indeed been grounded by the civil aviation authority, indefinitely. All planes had been cancelled, and I, along with thousands of other passengers, was now completely stranded in the terminal.

Worse still, I couldn't have my luggage back, as this was going to be flown to Durban separately from me! The loss of thousands of condoms wasn't my biggest problem though, as all my travellers cheques were in the case too, and I had only a limited amount of cash with me.

I spent the next two to three hours standing in queues, trying to find out more information and rescheduling a flight. Angry mobs were forming everywhere, and tempers were beginning to fray in the chaos which was getting out of control.

Hours later, I managed to rearrange another flight to Durban, but not until night time. Worse still, the airlines were greedily profit taking, and it cost me a small fortune to secure a ticket; money which would have been better spent on helping children.

The nuns had arranged to collect me from Durban earlier that day, but by now they must have heard news of the delays and driven the long distance back to Nkandla.

I was stranded in Johannesburg with only a few Rand left in my pocket. My lift had gone, my luggage too. It would be another eight hours before I could get on a plane, and not for the first time, my plans seemed in tatters, yet unbeknown to me, magic was about to happen.

With nothing else to do I went to a restaurant and sat down to collect my thoughts and get something to eat.

My meal soon came, but as I was eating, a well dressed black gentleman caught my eye as he walked towards me. The table next to me had just become available, yet for some reason he sat down next to me, and in impeccable English, asked if he could join me.

It seemed a bit odd at the time, but I nodded yes, and he started talking. At first he complained about the airport and the situation around us, then he talked about the weather and life generally, before the businessman, who had introduced himself as Vincent, asked me what had brought me to South Africa.

I still felt awkward telling people what I was doing, but he slowly dragged my story from me. He kept encouraging me to tell him more, and listened to my tales in astonishment. He told me about himself, and it turned out that he ran a large funeral business in Cape Town - but he was reaching despair at how many people he was burying each week, that had died from AIDS. Vincent had grown up through decades of apartheid, but had obviously become wealthy and successful since its end in the 1990's. It was obvious he longed to help the many children who were left behind as AIDS orphans - but he'd had no idea what he could do for them until now.

We continued to talk and Vincent seemed delighted to have met me. He paid for my lunch and then turned to me and pledged he would return to Cape Town and set up similar feeding schemes in schools there to help feed children!

It felt bizarre the way we met in the chaos of the day, but very gratifying to know this chance meeting may lead to thousands more children being fed each day.

Vincent's flight was due to leave long before mine, and we soon parted company, never to meet again. I guess I'll never know if he started feeding children in schools or not, but as odd as it sounds, our meeting didn't feel like an accident.

My rescheduled plane was due to fly at 8.00pm, but we did not begin to board it until after 9pm because of continuing delays. By now I had waited nearly twelve hours in the airport, and was beginning to feel the strain.

When I finally reached the boarding gate with my ticket, I handed it to the clerk, who tried to process it, before looking at me timidly. "It seems with all the problems of the day we have somehow double booked this seat, Sir, it's already taken." "Oh, you have to be joking", I exclaimed, just short of a shout. "I've paid hundreds of pounds for this ticket and sat around for twelve hours. I'm getting on that plane if I have to fly it myself," I said pointing out of the window.

"Wait here a moment, and I'll see what I can do for you," said the nervous clerk.

I waited impatiently, watching passenger after passenger board the plane, knowing there was going to be a major incident if anyone tried to stop me boarding this final flight to Durban for the night.

As the last passenger boarded, the clerk turned to me. "It looks like another passenger due on the flight isn't here, and I've just reallocated you their seat."

"Thank you", I said as my frustration slowly subsided.

I walked the short distance to the plane across the tarmac, then an almighty 'BANG' nearly dropped me to me knees. A thunderous sound ripped through the air, piecing my ears, as the heavens suddenly opened and bolts of lightning lit up the dark night sky above my head.

I bolted to the plane and shot up the stairs to safety. The waiting stewardess apologised profusely as she closed the cabin door behind me. "We won't be able to take off in this thunderstorm, I'm afraid, Sir. I'm sure it will pass over shortly and we'll be on our way soon. Let me show you to your seat."

I was shown to my reallocated seat and a smile spread across my face. It was a plush first class seat, which the missing passenger had kindly left behind, and as I sank back into the deep comfortable seat, I gave out a sigh.

I sat on the plane for another hour, sipping champagne and eating delicacies in the comfort of first class, until the storm eventually passed over. Then, finally, I was in the air and at last on my way to Durban.

As we flew, I knew Sister Hedwig was long gone, and that I would be stranded in the airport lounge for the night unless I could find my suitcase and my travellers cheques.

An hour later and I arrived in Durban to further scenes of chaos and had no idea where to go next - should I haul up here for the night and sleep on the floor until morning, or try and find my luggage in the anarchy of the airport?

I spotted a porter and went to ask him if he knew where uncollected luggage might be stored, or if even he even knew if any had come from across from Johannesburg that day.

"Hi," I said as I approached him. "Do you know where any uncollected luggage is kept? I've just arrived from Johannesburg and don't know where my case can be collected." The porter looked at me for a moment. "Are you Kevin Allen?" he said to my surprise. "Yes," I said, confused that he should even know my name. "I've been keeping your case safe all day," he said, as he led me to a small locked room with a single case sitting in it. "Wow, that was easy," I said to him in amazement. He smiled and nodded, and went back to his duties amid the chaos, as I was quickly reunited with my case of condoms, in a most unusual way!

I left the airport determined to find a cheap hotel for the night and get some rest before trying to find my way in to Nkandla in the morning.

I walked outside to more scenes of disarray and approached one of the taxi-drivers for a lift.

"Can you take me to a cheap hotel in Durban?" I asked the driver, pleased to have been able to commandeer him. "The Hilton Hotel," he replied. "No, not the Hilton, just a cheap hotel close to the airport if you know of any," I said. "Oh, sorry no, I'm waiting to take a passenger to the Hilton Hotel – my friend over there will help you."

He pointed to one of his colleagues, whistling to him loudly, as he pointed at me. The taxi driver acknowledged his friend, and I made my way towards him.

"Can you take me to a cheap hotel in Durban?" I said as I opened the cab door and started to climb in to his taxi. "No, no," he said to my frustration, "my friend here will take you," and he knocked on the roof of the next taxi, as the driver popped open the boot so I could put in my case.

Thankfully, this driver would take me and I climbed into his cab to my great relief. My chirpy driver was chatting happily, but I was exhausted and had been travelling across two days now, with little sleep.

"Can you take me to a cheap hotel, please?" I asked wearily. "Sure," he laughed, as we left the airport and headed into the night. He continued to chat happily, but I wasn't really listening, and he seemed content to talk to himself as much as to me.

It was dark in the taxi, but suddenly my senses began to tingle as I looked across to the driver. "Oh my God - David! Is that you? No way! Do you remember taking me into Zululand by taxi a few years ago to help me track down a young Zulu boy, and we stayed with the nuns?"

"Kevin!" he exclaimed in astonishment. "It's you, I can't believe it! I always knew I would see you again one day!"

I had first met David nearly three years ago on my first trip, and had taken such a profound journey with him then that we had a bond of friendship that went beyond words.

Nevertheless, it was simply, utterly incredible we were sitting next to each other again like this now. We talked as we drove and David laughed. "I think I am destined to be your personal taxi-driver whenever you come to Durban."

Destined indeed! David had undoubtedly saved my life all those years back, and I would never had found the nuns or Sne, or gone on to set up the fruit to school schemes without him.

I had written to him a few times over the years – but never knew if my letters had arrived – but David told me he had kept them all.

I just couldn't believe I had met him again in this way, it was simply unbelievable. David had only been working for an hour or so that night – and as with my first journey, I had delay after delay, and then I'd been redirected to him by other taxi drivers who wouldn't take my fare! He seemed to be there when I needed help most, and I simply couldn't explain how.

We carried on talking and I soon realised that David needed help himself now. He spoke softly with an unusual sadness, as he told me of his family, and how his sister had died of AIDS a year ago, leaving two young orphans in his care. He had taken in his nieces, and was now forced to work extra shifts to help pay to bring up his extended family.

I had promised David long ago that one day we would met again, and that I would help him; and here, now, the fates had brought us back together again.

We pulled up to the hotel and David called the porter and told him to take good care of me. The porter nodded in acknowledgement and went to the boot for my case. As we were getting out of the car I glanced at the cab clock for the time. It was 11.11pm! I just burst out laughing in almost madness. David couldn't have understood why I was laughing, or known that I saw these numbers daily, but he looked at me smiling, "They are magical numbers, Kevin."

Magic or miracle, chance or coincidence, meeting David in this way again really blew my mind.

But I wasn't even in Zululand yet, and this was only the start of another incredible journey…

Causing a Kerfuffle

I'd arranged to meet David the next morning for a lift back to the airport.

As he dropped me off, I was able to give him some much needed cash to help him through the tough times he was facing. Words aren't needed in situations like this, and David didn't seem to know whether to laugh or cry! Just looking at his face sent me into fits of laughter, and he burst out laughing too. We hugged in a way which transcended words, and I felt a deep humbleness engulf me.

As he drove away, all I could do was smile, knowing our paths would surely cross again in the future – and I would help him fulfil his dreams of owning his own taxi one day if I could.

I knew the nuns wouldn't abandon me in Durban, and no sooner had I trundled into the airport with my case, I spotted Hedwig talking with another nun.

"Hey stranger," I said as I sneaked up behind her. "Kevin!" she cried, smiling. "I thought we had lost you!" Hedwig's words hit a chord with me. Back home I would get lost just trying to find my way around Liverpool, yet here for some reason, I always found my way.

Sister hugged me and introduced me to her companion for the day, Sister Constance.

Sister Constance was one of those people who you could immediately connect with, and she smiled at me laughing playfully, "Hello Banana Man.".

"Don't start with that," I said, as Sister Hedwig looked on, knowing I was still uncomfortable with my adopted name. "Let me take your case Kevin, the car is this way." "OK," I said as I followed them.

"So what have you brought for us this time, more clothes and toys for the children?" asked Hedwig. "I'll show you later," I said bashfully, not quite sure how to tell the nuns I'd brought thousands of condoms for them!

It was a glorious day and the sun shimmered endlessly on the ocean as we drove up the beautiful South African coastline for mile after mile, before heading inland en route to Nkandla. I talked with Hedwig and Constance as we travelled, and they were like two peas in a pod. They had been allowed to stay out for the night, to wait for me in Durban, and were like little children who had been allowed to stay off school for the day, and obviously enjoying the rare freedom.

As we headed deeper inland the scenery began to change as the traffic thinned to a trickle. Large shops and luxury homes gradually turned to shacks and huts, as the cars made way for shoeless children wandering the dirt tracks, which stretched on for miles.

Before long, small groups of children appeared at makeshift roadside stalls, trying to sell fruit for a pittance of a living, and Sister didn't ask questions when I told her to pull over again and again to buy their produce.

Time after time happy faces appeared at the car window, thrusting fruit towards me in desperation of a sale of a few pence. Each time we drove off, we would leave to the sight of children dancing and waving in the road, each having just received a handful of banknotes, in return for a banana, an apple or an orange.

The Sisters found this hilarious, and it was funny to watch the children as their faces lit up. But this was the reason I had returned here, and it was heartbreaking too. Although I had managed to maintain the fruit schemes, I hadn't been in Africa for nearly a year now, and soon felt more alive than I had for the past twelve months.

"Kevin always shops this way," Hedwig explained to Constance as we continued to stop and buy more and more fruit. Before long the car filled with the familiar smells of fresh pineapple and mango, banana and orange - and it wasn't long before we were stopping again, this time passing out the fruit we had bought, and feeding hungry children by the dozen.

The day had been long, but passed quickly, and by the time we reached Nkandla, the hour was late.

As we drove into town, it seemed to have changed on the surface, with more municipal buildings being built, a small play area, and bigger shops and market place. A small bank had even appeared which was helping the people access government grants now.

"Wow, things really look like they are changing for the better," I said to Sister. "A little," she replied sadly, "but most of it is superficial and the people are still suffering greatly."

We soon entered the sanctuary of the convent and I was quickly welcomed by the nuns. How I'd forged such a close bond with them, I don't know. They knew I had no interest in Catholicism, yet still welcomed me warmly.

Hedwig showed me to the dining room to get a drink, as more nuns came to welcome me back with a loving hug. As they did an older nun entered the room, whom I had not previously met. Hedwig spoke with her for a brief moment and then introduced me to her. "This is Kevin from England," she said politely as the nun approached me to shake my hand. "I haven't been travelling for two days for a handshake," I said smiling, as I ignored her hand and grabbed her for a hug. I hadn't noticed the atmosphere in the room had changed slightly, but as I embraced her I caught sight of Hedwig who was turning white with horror at my actions. Hedwig looked at me, shaking her head, gesturing 'NO', as I continue to hug the nun, who wasn't responding in kind.

I smiled in bemusement, then dread set in as I realised I had somehow breached an unknown protocol. I slowly let go of the nun who faced me down blankly. "Hello Kevin," she said politely, as she brushed herself off and composed herself.

"Hello," I beamed back with a cheeky smile to try and break the tension, before she turned away and left the room. I looked at Hedwig and threw her a puzzled glance.

"Kevin, sit with me for a moment," she said. I sank into the seat like a naughty child about to be told off, knowing I had somehow done wrong. "This sister is the Superior General of our church and travels Africa and Europe inspecting our convents. She is here to assess us at the moment and will decide which convent we will stay at over the coming years.

"This means any of us could be reposted to another convent today, even overseas. We are having a meeting with her tonight to find out our fate, and all the sisters here are on edge today, and worried they might be moved elsewhere."

I hadn't realised the nuns had such a high ranking figurehead who controlled their lives in this way. I had just hugged tight one of the most revered women of the Catholic Church, and it was probably the first physical contact she'd had with a man in over half a century!

"Sorry," I said, feeling guilty for my innocent actions, knowing if the gods existed, they were surely watching me again, and shaking the heavens with roars of laughter.

"Kevin, let me show you to your room. You can leave your suitcase here if you like and I will unpack the things you have brought for our poor children." No I better take it with me for now," I said in panic of creating more chaos. "I'll see you tomorrow with Sister Ellen and show you what I've brought then."

I'd only been in Nkandla for five minutes and I was already causing a kerfuffle!

Empire

I was shown to my room and decided I better keep the condoms to myself for the time being. It's not every day you find yourself in a convent in the middle of Africa, scurrying around a room, hiding thousands of loose condoms in the wardrobes. But then people were dying in Zululand, and here I was worrying about the finer points of convent politics. Besides, it almost seemed normal to find myself in these kinds of situations nowadays.

I relaxed for the rest of the evening in privacy and sat spellbound as the sun began to set. Deep bursts of colour broke through the thin veil of cloud, as the sky shone red and orange, purple and violet. I sat watching until twilight fell, then through to darkness as the stars peppered the night sky, as if just for me.

In the morning I woke early and went to find the Sisters, who were in the dining area sipping tea, and chatting happily between themselves. "The meeting went well last night?" I asked Hedwig. "Yes," she whispered. "We are all safe! But I have to take our Mother to the next convent she is assessing today, so you can come with me as it's a long drive."

I had hoped to avoid the Mother General after our intimate encounter yesterday, and had really wanted to spend the day visiting families and hungry children with food parcels. Now I would be trapped in a car with Mother for hours…and worse still, Hedwig was driving!

I ate little as Hedwig arranged for me to meet her outside in half an hour for our road trip. "I'm looking forward to it," I sighed as I left her.

It was a typically hot African day as I walked the short distance to the car. As I approached, Hedwig was giggling with her new best friend Constance. "What are you pair up to now?" I smiled as I saw them. "Its nuns' talk," they said, without saying more.

'Mother' was already seated in the back of the car, so I darted for the front passenger seat, so as not to be stuck in the back with her all day. Constance saw my move - but she was too late.

"Beat you," I grinned, as I cast her a smile, and she cast me a frown, knowing she had drawn the short straw for the day, and looking unimpressed that she would have to entertain Mother for the duration of the drive.

We were soon travelling into the vast Zulu countryside, and I found myself transfixed by the scenery as I gazed at the homesteads which speckled the hills. Hedwig was transfixed too, but to the road, and would squeal with delight as she swerved at the last moment to avoid the free roaming cattle which wandered the road without fear. Constance meanwhile was trying her best to make polite conversation with Mother General, and I knew she must have been thinking unholy thoughts of me because of her burden.

I waved and smiled to the children we passed on the roadside, as we travelled ever onwards. The children always smiled and waved back excitedly, and it was amazing to witness their friendliness despite their awful plight. We kept driving and I didn't have a clue where we were until Hedwig pointed down a track. "Look, Kevin, that road leads to Rorkes Drift. I must take you there one day so you can see where the British and Zulus once fought."

I had long been trying to piece together the historical jigsaw puzzle of events which had brought the Zulus to their knees, and had tracked back their problems to the Anglo-Zulu war of 1879, and the now famous battles of Rorkes Drift and Isandlwana.

The war had been an illegal and unwarranted act of British aggression against the Zulus. Illegal because it was encouraged by Queen Victoria at the height of her imperial reign, yet it was never authorised by parliament, who fully opposed it.

Rural Zululand couldn't have changed much in the last 150 years, and I found my mind drifting back in time, as I imagined the sight of the thousands of British troops wearily marching up the road I now travelled. Ox drawn wagons laboured under the heavy burden of supplies, as columns of soldiers marched to war, commanded by officers riding their stallions of status.

In my mind's eye I saw a fortified camp take shape with typical military efficiency; then watched on as the British marched deep into the hills, in murderous pursuit of the Zulu. But the Zulus relied on deception and surprise, and had tricked the advancing army with a ruse. As the British marched onwards, twenty thousand Zulu warriors had amassed to attack the British base camp at Isandlwana.

I visualised the Zulu as they silently surrounded the camp under camouflage of the countryside, before they swarmed off the hills in wave after wave. As they did, the sound of the blood-curdling charge transcended time, piecing my ears, and the hairs on the back of my neck stood on end, as I relived the melee in my mind's eye.

All around me I could see, hear and feel the panic and chaos, with the sounds of dying screams echoing across the ages, as men were shot, speared and slain in a vicious bloody battle. The riffle shots, with puffs of white smoke, just weren't heavy enough to halt the aggressive fighting spirit and raw courage of the Zulu - and the lush green grass soon ran red with blood.

In these dreadful moments of history thousands died. Over 1,300 well armed British troops were slain by the spear, and the Zulu lost a thousand men to the bullet and the bayonet.

But the Zulus weren't finished fighting for their Kingdom yet. Fired up by victory, they broke away into bands, with thousands marching onwards to Rorkes Drift. Beating their shields with spears to frighten their enemy, the Zulus swarmed towards the small outpost, held by just 145 terrified men. Ferocious fighting erupted, and corpses piled high in a battle which finally left the Zulus defeated by the gun.

After the battle no Zulu was spared, no prisoners taken. Five hundred wounded Zulus were ruthlessly executed, in an atrocity hidden from history, but which typified the Imperial attitude towards those they conquered.

As the Zulus fell in battle, I saw desperate young children left in the valleys. Orphaned by fate and left homeless, hungry, frightened and alone.

The car jolted violently as we hit a pothole, bringing me abruptly out of my daydream. I glared out of the car window and saw desperate young children left in the valleys. Orphaned by fate and left homeless, hungry, frightened and alone.

Hedwig looked at me. "Are you OK, Kevin?"
I looked back briefly "Yes," I replied…but I wasn't.

Nothing had changed in Zululand in over a century – and it had been my ancestors, my countrymen, my queen, who had brought the mighty Zulu nation to their knees. And they had never recovered, not even to this day.

"A very remarkable people, the Zulu. They defeat our generals; they convert our bishops; they have settled the fate of a great European dynasty."

Benjamin Disraeli

Beyond Belief

By now my mood had changed and I wanted to get out of the car and start feeding children by the roadside again. I put on my headphones and turned up the volume to try and drown out the madness of the world, to the deafening thud of club anthems.

We continued to drive for an age, deeper and deeper into nowhere, until we eventually arrived at the convent at the foot of a mountain, in an area of immense natural beauty.

I was glad to get out of the car after my trip back through time – and we were soon greeted by the waiting nuns, who were expecting our arrival anxiously.

The convent's sister superior was a beautiful person and we chatted for a few minutes as I stretched my legs. Then she introduced me to one of her friends, a Jesuit priest who had arrived just a few hours earlier. Sister explained Edward had travelled from Zimbabwe in desperation of obtaining supplies for his local community.

He was a large white man and a larger than life character, who was incredibly sprightly for his eighty-six years of age. As we spoke he picked up on my accent, and to my astonishment asked me if I was from Liverpool.

"Yes!" I said, shocked he had ever even heard of Liverpool. "Well actually I live over the other side of the river Mersey nowadays, on the Wirral."

He looked at me smiling with delight. "I've lived in Zimbabwe for well over forty years now," he said "but originally I came from Rock Ferry on the Wirral…do you watch Tranmere Rovers play football?"

"No way!" I said as a shiver ran through me – "you come from Rock Ferry and liked Tranmere Rovers!"

Rock Ferry is a tiny area of Birkenhead about a mile square in size, and I had lived there most of my life.

Edward reminisced for a while and I soon discovered that he had been brought up only a few roads away from the home that I had sold, which had helped start the fruit to school schemes in Nkandla a few years earlier!

Edward spoke with a glint of magic in his eyes as he revealed his deepest desire these last few years had been to get a message to his sister in the UK, to tell her he was still alive and well.

Incredibly, she still lived in Rock Ferry too – and when he passed me her address I saw she lived less than a minute's drive from where I lived now!

As the situation started to sink in I began laughing to myself, then spontaneously with Edward, knowing the fates were in motion once more, as they had been so many times in this incredible land of mysteries. Only four days earlier I had been standing in Rock Ferry – Edward in Zimbabwe. Now in the middle of southern Africa, in the depths of Zululand, as far away from civilisation as one could imagine, I was talking to a man who had lived just two roads away from my home in times gone by. His greatest wish, his deepest desire, was to get a message to his sister in England – and by powers I don't try to explain, she lived within shouting distance of me. Not only that, but he had arrived at the retreat only hours before me, and if either of us had travelled any other day we would never have met.

It was beyond belief; but more than that, it was beyond chance.

We went for lunch and I chatted with Edward, fascinated with his tales of adventure stretching longer than I'd been alive. He had been helping children since before I was born, but as he spoke it became clear life in Zimbabwe was dire.

The currency had effectively collapsed because inflation was out of control, with a staggering rate of 200 million percent! Crops had failed, the government too. Infrastructure was disintegrating, especially healthcare and education. Ageing President Robert Mugabe, who had ruled the country with an iron fist for nearly three decades, was still clinging to power, and electoral fraud was rife.

Rhodesia, as the country was formerly known, had once been under colonial rule just like South Africa. Mugabe had at first been a liberating hero when he brought back rule to black people; he was even knighted by the Queen during an official visit to Britain in 1994! But now he was a tyrant, plain and simple, and guilty of human rights violations and economic genocide which was bringing his country to its knees.

As I listened to Edward I knew he did all he could to help the desperate people in the town where he worked, but it was clear he was fighting a losing battle.

After lunch I rejoined Hedwig and Constance, who were keen to give me a guided tour of the convent, and the tranquillity of the retreat was indescribable; suffice to say it was an oasis amid the pain and poverty surrounding it.

Hedwig seemed at peace as we walked, until we passed a newly rebuilt outhouse. She was visibly shaken as we approached it and her voice shook as she spoke. "This building was used as a hospice for the sick, but the straw roof caught fire, when one of the patients smoked a cigarette. One of our sisters, Sister Anne, lost her life trying to save the elderly patients. She had helped save five people, but went back into the burning building to try and save more." I knew from Hedwig's emails that Sister Anne had died trying to save the last three patients trapped in the hospice - and was only thirty-five when she had lost her life to the flames.

"There is so much sadness here already," Hedwig continued, "then a dreadful thing like this happens and it makes no sense – but God has his plan." I nodded in agreement, but I wasn't so sure, and I knew the fire had killed Sister Anne on Palm Sunday of all days.

We continued to walk through the idyllic gardens as we walked close to a small lake, where I caught sight of something moving and pointed to the distant bank. "What on earth is that?" I asked as I stared. Constance froze for a moment as the creature spotted us, before disappearing from sight. "I think it was a large crocodile or a komodo dragon," said Constance, backing away in almost a run. I followed her quickly, as did Hedwig, who was tugging on my tee-shirt playfully, pulling me back so she could pass first, and laughing as she did. "Are you scared, Kevin?" she laughed as she passed me giggling.

"Sometimes I forget I'm in Africa with all these creatures around me," I said as we paused and looked back. "Yes, you must get off the grass too and walk on the path, there are many poisonous snakes here." I jumped to the path in fright and turned to look to see if anything was slithering towards me! Hedwig burst out laughing with Constance. "Are you joking?" I asked, unsure. "No, you must be very careful here," they insisted, straight-faced, but I still wasn't sure if they were just playing a prank on me or not.

As we walked, the path began to narrow and Hedwig looked at me to see if I dared walk on the grass again. As she did I nudged her onto it. "Well, you reckon you're going to heaven and I'm going to hell, so I'm not talking any chances, the snakes can bite you instead," I said lightheartedly. Hedwig walked on the grass, strutting bravery to show no fear. As she did a large bee flew in her direction on her blindside. She could hear the buzz from behind her, but couldn't see the bee as it approached, and she screamed, running with Constance, as they flailed their arms in a panic. "Kevin, it's a bee, run!"

"I'm not falling for that," I said. "It's only a bee."

"It's an African bee, Kevin" I heard Constance cry as she disappeared at speed down the path towards a building. "Are they dangerous?" I shouted, but it was too late, they had fled.

Beauty and danger seemed to go hand-in-hand in this land, mixed with wonder and woe, and I froze as the bee flew by without showing its sting.

Hedwig and Constance were long gone by now, so I continued my walk alone and wandered into a secluded garden of intense beauty. I sat down and took in a deep breath, acknowledging the awe-inspiring nature which surrounded me, feeling overwhelmed by its splendour.

As I sat in awe, I was drawn to the incredible beauty of a flower and sat mesmerised by it for a moment. Then I experienced one of the most bizarre events of my life. It was an amazing experience and a deeply personal one, which was experienced in feelings, not words, making it difficult to describe, other than to say it left me with deep feelings that all things in nature were bound together as one.

I walked out of the garden in a bit of a daze, still pondering my surreal experience and wondering if I'd just had a lucid daydream, some sort of vision, or hallucinated in the heat!

I tracked down Hedwig, but didn't know how to tell her about my amazing experience in the garden, so said nothing.

Soon, it was time to leave Mother General to her duties, and set off on the long drive to back Nkandla before darkness fell. And I left in awe of this incredible land, called Zulu.

The Cradle of Life

Africa was often described as the cradle of life, and I had yet to come here without experiencing extraordinary events, and yesterday had been no exception.

Today, however, I was to visit Sne and Mbali again, and the Lindiwe family and the Petros' homestead too, and I was excited at the prospect.

But first I needed to visit more schools to explore the possibility of starting fruit projects there as another charity and the local Government had recently started feeding the children at Phalane.

At first I couldn't understand why the charity had begun feeding in Phalane. I was already feeding the children there with fruit, and there must have been tens of thousands of other children in different schools who needed food, so why double up at Phalane? It soon became clear that it was a political move, and it seemed the large charity didn't want some guy from Merseyside feeding a thousand children a day, whilst they fed none – and I suspected they wanted to oust me.

Whatever their intentions, this was brilliant news for me, and meant I could withdraw from Phalane and divert my resources to other schools. Instead of ousting me, the charity and government were inadvertently helping me expand my feeding schemes, without me having to find a penny extra!

Hedwig had drawn up a list of ten possible schools where we could move our schemes to, and the only sad thing for me was that I couldn't start feeding at them all.

The first school we visited was Nkandla High, a small school in the heart of the town, and one within a five minute drive of the convent. As we pulled up it looked like any other first world school from the outside, but like so much of South Africa, if you scratched under the surface a little, you found a different truth.

"How many children attend here?" I asked Hedwig as we arrived. "Five hundred, I think, but we will confirm this with the teachers," she replied as we got out of the car and walked into the grounds.

Racism had always been a strange concept to me. I had always seen people as people, children as children – and I judged people by their actions not their colour. Yet I was often reminded in Nkandla that I was white, and that I stood out like a sore thumb because of my colour.

Today was no different, and no sooner had I entered the school, when I became the centre of attention for the children. It wasn't long before I had an ever growing group of youngsters following me out of curiosity. I smiled and waved to them, but realised through their innocent attention, how uncomfortable life must be for so many people, simply because of the colour of their skin or the way they looked. I suppose we are all prisoners of our bodies in one way or another; none of us had any say before we were born in our colour, or our sex, our shape or our size, or any of our outward appearance.

Thinking about it, we didn't even have any choice in the country we were born in – let alone the time in history. I'd always considered myself pretty much in control of my life, but in reality, I was a slave to circumstance, just like everyone else.

I stayed close to Hedwig as we navigated our way through the school's corridors, until we found the headmaster's office. After a short introduction Sister explained to him that I was from England and had been running feeding schemes for some years at Phalane, and now wanted to help feed the children at his school. He seemed very excited by the proposal and was soon shaking my hand in gratitude. "Thank you, Banana Man," he said, grinning widely with delight, as I resigned myself to the fact I would be now be known by my pseudonym to hundreds more children.

We were given a grand tour of the school, and I agreed to start the schemes immediately.

We soon left Nkandla High and headed out of town to find the second school on Hedwig's list, Mttiyaqhwa High. "This school is similar to Phalane in size and has just under 950 children attending it," Hedwig said as we pulled up in a cloud of dust. "It is a good school and run by the town's mayor."

Break time was over at Mttiyaqhwa by the time we arrived so we quickly found the headmaster's office and introduced ourselves to one of the staff. The headmaster wasn't there at the time, so we talked with the deputy head, and the same scene as earlier quickly played out. Ten minutes later and we had repeated our success at

Nkandla High, and established a fruit programme for the children here too.

After our obligatory tour of the school we jumped back in the car in high spirits. "That was easy," I said to Hedwig as we drove away. "You should be pleased, Kevin. As well as the thousand children at Phalane, fifteen hundred more children will be fed at school each day now."

"Another charity has been feeding at four other schools for over a year now, and Catholics from America have said they will start feeding at a school with 900 children in it next year too."

I looked out of the window, smiling, knowing that as usual, what was transpiring here had little to do with me, but delighted that the feeding schemes were starting to ripple outwards, helping thousands more children than I could ever hope to feed alone. My greatest hope now was that the large charity and government would follow my lead again, and set up new feeding programmes at Nkandla High and Mttiyaqhwa High. If that happened I could divert my resources again, and feed another 1,500 children daily without having to find any additional funding!

Hedwig could sense my happiness, "Let us return to the convent now. We will visit Sne and the other families this afternoon, and you can buy them some gifts from town before we see them if you like."

Although I kept track of Sne via email with the sisters, I hadn't seen him in nearly a year, and Hedwig's suggestion to shop for gifts from town had by mind buzzing with what I could buy for him.

Zulu children were mad about football, and Sne was no exception. His dream was to become a professional footballer one day, and like most Zulu children, played at every opportunity he could. Mbali's dream was to become a stewardess, as she had wanted to know all the places people went on planes, and must have held deep and exciting memories of her trip to England, a few years ago.

The town had expanded greatly since my last visit – but it was still very limited in what it had to offer as far as gifts went.

"There is a secondhand clothes shop in town," Hedwig said as we drove the short distance to the shops. It didn't sound very appealing at first, but as we entered the store I noticed it had some secondhand football shirts for sale.

"Let's get him a football shirt," I said as I rummaged through the neatly displayed shirts. The stock was limited, and expensive too given the local economy, and I could see how highly prized foreign football shirts were here. I was looking for an England shirt, but couldn't see any – but then found a Liverpool top with GERRARD written on the back! "Hey, Sister look at this, this is where I come from - do you think it will fit Sne?"

"No, it's too small for him," replied Hedwig. "He's growing up fast now – what about this one?" Hedwig held up a Brazil shirt which looked as good as new. "Are they a good football team?" she asked.

"Yeah, they're not bad," I said, laughing to myself, knowing Sne was going to love it!

"We'll take this one please," I said to the storekeeper, who was by now rubbing his hands together in anticipation of the sale of such a highly valued top.

By the time we left the store I had caught the shopping bug, and took Hedwig on a mini shopping spree to spend some money on the children in the small selection of shops the town had, knowing each purchase was going to delight them, whilst helping the local traders too.

It wasn't long before the car was brimming with goods – and we had even found a radio, a much prized gift for Mbali.

As we drove to Sne's homestead, Hedwig told me that the original documentary makers had sent money to the sisters to help build a house for Sne and Mbali last year. "That's fantastic news!" I said with delight.

Sne and Mbali were both in boarding schools now and doing well with their studies. During the holidays they returned to stay with their uncle Simon and his family, but had been living in traditional mud huts, which were run down and basic, to say the least.

The stone house which had been built for them at the homestead had a secure front door, windows, running water and electricity, and was a huge asset for ones so young.

Before the home had been built, Sne and Mbali had to walk over quarter of a mile to there nearest stream for water and carry it back in huge buckets, which would be no small feat for a grown man, let alone children!

The car bounced along the dusty track as we drew ever nearer to Sne's homestead, and I hoped the children would be happy with the gifts we'd brought.

As we pulled up, two faces appeared at the door and I saw Sne smiling as we climbed out the car to greet them. It was incredible to see them both again, and I couldn't believe how fast they were growing up now, especially Mbali who was rapidly becoming a young lady.

They proudly showed me around their new home - and no sooner had Sne caught sight of the football shirt, then he put it on and started running around with his football. And that was that; so we spent the next fifteen minutes playing football in the African heat, until I could run no more. By now Mbali had seen her radio, and was listening to music like any normal teenager could.

We'd brought the children loads more gifts and enough food to keep them fed for months!

I knew the children were both doing well at school with their studies, but they of course had no source of income, and I'd brought money for Mbali so she could buy some essentials for herself and Sne for the year ahead.

The smiles which broke across the children's faces as they realised they had money was amazing – and despite the terrible life they had endured, I knew in that moment that they were the lucky ones.

We chatted and played for a while longer, but time was always my enemy here. All too soon we had to leave, and like a prisoner seeing his family briefly on visiting day, I was soon parted from the children again.

But I knew I still had vital work to do here today, and I had a very important appointment with a special little girl, Nobuhtle, whose name meant 'beautiful one'. Nobuhtle was one of Lindiwe's daughters and I had always seemed to miss her on my previous trips. Yet I knew from Hedwig she was struggling badly with the sickness of her mother, and she'd already lost her father to AIDS many years ago.

Zulu society was very matriarchal and a great burden fell to Nobuhtle as Lindiwe's eldest daughter. She had lived a truly terrible life these last years and was left to look after her siblings alone when her mother was too sick to care for them. At one time Hedwig had thought Nobuhtle had AIDS herself and had pushed Lindiwe to take her to hospital for a test. But it was a three mile walk to the hospital, and some days Lindiwe struggled to get out of bed, let alone walk a six mile round trip journey. Worse still, the hospital wasn't free and the government charged a user's fee in this decimated community, rife with poverty.

Eventually, Lindiwe had raised enough money and strength to take Nobuhtle to hospital, and thankfully she tested negative for AIDS.

Yet Nobuhtle still struggled each day as she watched her mum dying slowly of AIDS, and went to bed each night not knowing if her mother would be alive in the morning. Lindiwe had told her that on her death she was not to panic, but to find Hedwig as she would know what to do. This was a great burden to Nobuhtle - and to Hedwig too. So many people relied on Hedwig for help and I could feel her buckling under the pressure. Lindiwe had told Hedwig that on her death someone would come and help her children. "Who will come?" Hedwig had replied to her, knowing no one was going to come here and help.

I knew who would come for Lindiwe's children when that fateful moment arrived; but gladly that was my burden for another day.

Today I had come for a different reason – to bring a glimmer of happiness to Nobuhtle, and to let here know people did care about her and her family.

Lindiwe's homestead was only about a mile away from Sne's home, and it wasn't long before we arrived. I walked the steep climb down the hillside, weighed down with the goods I was carrying, but smiling with each step I took.

As we approached Lindiwe's house, Hedwig called to the children to let them know we were coming, and I put the bags of food and clothes on the floor outside the house to catch my breath. We knocked on the door and a young girl opened it then ran towards me and threw her arms around me, clinging tight.

This was an emotionally charged moment which took me a little by surprise. "Hello again," I said as I looked down smiling at her as she clung on, a little shocked she should even remember me from my previous trips. 'Busy Bee' whom I'd met on my first trip remembered me too – he was taller now, but we were soon playing football again.

Hedwig was talking to the children in Zulu by now, and greeted them with loving hugs of her own, before sending them out to collect the bags of food we had brought. Hungry children don't need telling twice, and they shot out of the house to find the food.

Nobuhtle was a young teenager and a little shyer than her younger siblings, but I paid her special attention as I gave her the gifts we had bought for her from town. As the children tucked into bananas, I passed them sweets and balloons, and some clothes and toys. I'd brought money for Lindiwe too, but she had gone to town for some much needed supplies, so I split the money between the children, who proceeded to run around waving it in the air as if they had just won the lottery!

Hedwig thought it hilarious as they ran around the homestead in delight. I knew Lindiwe would have her hands full trying to get the cash back off them, but I had brought it to help her children, and it was a funny to watch their reactions.

Besides, I'd only given the youngsters a few pounds each, and gave charge of the balance to Nobuhtle, as her face lit up with delight.

We stayed for a while and I played with the children while Hedwig assessed their health. As we left, the children ran up the hillside to wave us off, and we were soon on the road again to our final destination; Petros.

Of all the men I had met in my life, I held Petros as one of the kindest. He had nothing in the world; not wealth nor income, opportunity nor education. He lived in a simple mud hut without power or water, and had experienced hardship daily in his life. He had lived through decades of apartheid, and watched catastrophic pandemics decimate his community. He must have felt hunger more times than a person should, and thirsted often for change. Yet despite it all he had retained his humour and his humanity, and still found the will to share his life and his love with the desperate children around him.

We pulled up to the Petros homestead and Hedwig beeped her horn to alert the family to our presence. The children ran to greet us and helped us carry the provisions we had brought them, as Petros and Irene came to see what all the fuss was about.

I gave the children balloons and sweets, and as usual you would have thought it was Christmas by their reactions. Petros appeared from his hut and despite the fact he spoke no English, and I no Zulu, we were soon laughing and joking together in a language of our own.

I always carried a spare t-shirt with me and couldn't believe my luck as I rummaged to the bottom of my backpack. I remembered how Petros had cherished my England cap last time we'd met, and in town how valued foreign football shirts were here. I pulled my

England top from my back pack and passed it to Petros, who held it for a second just looking at it, before a wide smile spread across his face as he realised it was for him.

"Tell him I brought it all the way from England especially for him," I told Hedwig. I hadn't of course, and I was sorry to see it go, but as Hedwig relayed my message, I knew Petros felt special and he would treasure the shirt.

It was a tragedy of humanity that mankind didn't stand up against poverty and corruption, challenging those with power to change lives of those in desperate need.

To fulfill a man's dreams or make him feel special, to give a child food or to make them smile, to hand out fruit randomly to hungry people on the road. In truth, I'd never done a charitable thing in my life - just the right thing - and this seemed to generate something money couldn't buy: hope.

Despite the heat, clouds had been gathering all day, and as the heavens began to open, we said goodbye to Petros and the children and headed back to the convent before dusk fell.

Time flies

Land of the Free

The atmosphere at the convent had relaxed after the departure of Mother General the day before, and after a light meal I spent the rest of the evening drinking beer with the nuns and talking. I felt almost apologetic as I told them about the thousands of condoms I had in my room, which I had brought to help them in their fight against AIDS.

Despite my slight embarrassment, Sister Ellen seemed pleased that she had access to them and could give them out as a precautionary measure to young couples, and I felt a lot better that my efforts to get them here hadn't been in vain.

As the night progressed I arranged with Hedwig that we would go to the orphanage in the morning, before heading out of town to feed more children. My strength was slowly waning as the hours passed and I was still struggling to recover from the long inbound journey. Yet it was my last day here tomorrow, and I would have to travel back home, so I retired to bed and soon fell into a deep sleep.

In the morning I woke with a bang, as Hedwig knocked loudly on my door to see were I was. "Kevin, are you ready to go? It's 10 o'clock."

Startled and disoriented, I tried to gain my bearings as I poked my head over the blankets. "I'll be with you in five minutes" I shouted, squinting in the brightness of the sun which poured into the room. "OK," said Hedwig, "I'll wait for you by the car." The sisters got up at an unholy hour every day to pray and sing hymns, usually at around

4am – but Hedwig didn't know I was suffering from jet lag.

I climbed out of bed wearily and went to shower, knowing I'd soon be wide awake whether I wanted to be or not. The shower in my room hadn't been working since I had arrived and I had been getting freezing cold showers each morning just to try and stay clean and wash away some of the grime. "God, that's FREEZING," I cried as I turned on the taps and stepped under the ice cold water.

I jumped out of the shower as fast as I had jumped in through the shock of the cold. Shivering, I dried off as quickly as I could and threw on a pair of shorts and walked outside so the sun could warm my skin.

"That's better," I sighed as I stood there enjoying the heat for a moment, then grabbed my t-shirt and my backpack, and ran to meet Hedwig at the car. "Do you want to get something to eat before we go?" Hedwig asked. "No, I'm fine," I said as I mustered a sleepy smile and yawned involuntarily. "I'll get some fruit from town later after we've been to the orphanage."

Hedwig nodded as we got into the car to drive the short distance to the orphanage. Despite my cold shower, my head was still foggy with sleep and I could have happily curled up like one of the cats at the convent and slept on the floor in the sunlight. By now Hedwig was singing a hymn to herself, and I rolled down my window to release the noise and let in the sounds of the world outside.

We soon arrived at the orphanage and I got out of the car and stretched. I released a final loud yawn to shake off my tiredness as I noticed the resident dog tied up in a kennel. I had first met the dog a few years ago as an energetic pup who bounded around endlessly, but today he looked terrified as I approached him cautiously. "What's wrong with the dog?" I asked Hedwig as I coaxed him towards me. Hedwig laughed sheepishly to disguise her guilt "Oh my God, that poor dog. I was leaving the convent the other week and reversed over him by accident. We had to call the vet and thankfully he was OK, but I don't think he likes me anymore!"

"No. You didn't!" I exclaimed, knowing full well the hazards of Hedwig's driving.

I stroked him sympathetically for a minute and gave him some words of wisdom on how to best avoid Hedwig in the future, knowing he understood every word I whispered.

As we continued into the grounds, we found thirty children playing happily in the gardens, and as each saw Hedwig they ran to her for a hug. It was ironic that as a nun Hedwig would never have children, yet she had still become a loving mother to so many.

As usual I had bought some small gifts, sweets and balloons for the children and gave them out as an excited furour erupted all around me.

After this we sat in the garden for a while and played with the children, before Hedwig gave me a tour of the orphanage.

"It is sad for me that I can look after so few children here, when the need is so great," said Hedwig, who only had places for a maximum of thirty children at any one time. We walked through the large vegetable garden which had been planted to help feed the children, and as we did I realised food grown in this way was free.

Then I noticed a large piece of vacant land behind the orphanage, fenced off. "Who owns this?" I asked curiously. "It belongs to the sisters," Hedwig said. "Wow, that must be at least three or four acres, you could easily build a second orphanage or child village there," I said as I surveyed the land purposefully. "Yes, I would like to," nodded Hedwig in agreement, "but I do not have the means to do such a thing."

"If I could raise the money for a second orphanage would you let me build one here?" I asked excitedly. "Yes of course, Kevin; you can do this?" "Sure," I replied, not having the faintest idea if I could. "How much do you think it would cost to build another orphanage here?" I continued. "The one you see here is large and was very expensive, costing about £12,500," she said sadly.

£12,500 was about 200,000 Rand, an absolute fortune in these parts, and in truth Hedwig had no hope of ever raising this kind of money to expand the orphanage further. But in my economy it was a realistic enough sum to raise.

I looked at the land and at the vegetable gardens again. "This land could even be used to grow fruit on to give to out at the schools. We could feed many more children this way." "Yes," replied Hedwig.

"That would not be difficult to do either and I will speak to the sisters later, they will let you have this land if you can use it."

We left the orphanage and returned briefly to the convent to pick up Constance, then headed to town and cleared a stunned trader's stall of all her produce, before driving into the surrounding countryside to feed impoverished children.

"Many of the orphans play football in the fields up here," said Hedwig as we bumped along the dilapidated road. Sister knew the area well and it wasn't long before we found children and spent the rest of the day passing out fruit as we travelled.

On the journey back to the convent Sister pointed to a large homestead. "That is one of the Zulu chief's homes. He is a very important man in our community and owns all the land in Nkandla."

"What do you mean he owns all the land?" I laughed. "He owns it all," Hedwig repeated. "When people in the community need land to set up a homestead or to farm, they go to the chief, tell him why they need the land and it is his duty to decide if they can have it or not."

"But how do people pay for it?" I quizzed. Hedwig laughed at my ignorance. "They don't pay for it. It is free."

"Free! It's really free!" I said, still a little confused.
"Yes, of course it's free. It is for his people - the land he grants them is free."

My mind was working overtime by now. "Do you think he would give me a large piece of land to grow a fruit plantation on, to help feed the children at the schools?"

"He may do" replied Hedwig. "If he understands it will help the community I don't see why not. I can arrange for you to meet him next time you come to Nkandla if you like."

If I would like! "Yes I would" I replied, trying to restrain my excitement.

I still couldn't believe my ears. The land here was so abundant it was free; completely, absolutely free! It was controlled by the chief, who allocated it for the good of his people and he didn't charge them a penny for it.

We drove back to the convent and arrived just as the nuns were preparing for dinner. We walked into the dining room and I sat with Sister Ellen and Sister Eobarda, as Hedwig explained to them I would like the land at the back of the convent to build a second orphanage or plant with fruit. After a short discussion the sisters agreed. "Yes Kevin, the land is yours if you can put it to use."

Back home I owned no land or property of my own and still rented a house for my family after we had sold our own a few years earlier. Yet I had just been gifted a large piece of land for free, and may be given much more in the future, and my head was in a spin as to how I could best utilise it!

Time Flies

I went to bed that night thinking through all the incredible events which had occurred over the last few days, knowing tomorrow it was time to return home after another mind blowing journey of self-discovery.

I woke early in the morning and packed my near empty case and went to find the nuns to say goodbye.

The nuns had gathered to meet me, and after a small breakfast, they gave me numerous craft gifts which Sister Sola had made with the local Zulu women.

Of all the sisters, sister Sola was one of my favourites. She must have been well into her eighties; her hearing was failing, her memory too. Physically she was small and frail - yet the energy which flowed through her was immense and I had connected with her deeply at heart.

I hugged her tight and told her she would see me again, then hugged the others too - before having a photograph with them all, as they blessed me on my journey home.

I always found it strange to receive the blessing of the nuns, but it was nice in its own way, and I knew they prayed for me too, which I still find bizarre to this day.

Hedwig was to drive me back to the airport, and I was glad of this as it would allow us more time to talk before I left her again.

It was a hot day, but we were engrossed in conversation most of the drive back, and despite the length of the journey, time passed quickly. We had to stop for petrol after a while, and as Hedwig filled up the tank, I went into the garage and found they were selling cold cans of Red Bull, so bought two.

"Hey Sister, try this," I said as I returned to the car. "It's called Red Bull and it gives you wings," I joked. Hedwig looked at me blankly. "It helps you stay awake when you're feeling tired," I explained as I sipped my drink.

Hedwig had never tasted anything like it before and quickly emptied her can to quench her thirst, before we hit the road again.

"You like it then, I take it" I laughed. "Yes, it is very nice, Kevin" said Hedwig.

Unfortunately Sister had never experienced a 'caffeine hit' before, and she soon began to drive erratically and chatter noticeably louder!

"Oh God" I thought, as we swerved at the last minute, barely missing a troop of monkeys which had darted across the road in front of us, as sister laughed aloud! I might as well have given her drugs, I thought to myself as I tightened my seatbelt and gripped the door handle to steady myself.

The rest of the drive back to Durban was a little intense, but as we arrived safely at the airport, Hedwig was starting to come down a little. "What was that drink called, Kevin?" Sister asked as she escorted me to the check-in. "Red Bull - but you should only drink one a day if you're not used to them," I said, as I imagined the chaos I had unleashed on the world and trying not to laugh.

Soon after this, Sister waved me off once more – and I knew I would return as soon as I could. I had done much this trip, yet I felt incomplete.

Twenty-six uncomfortable hours later I arrived back home to the great relief of Joanne and my children. I knew Joanne still worried each time I journeyed to Africa, but she knew why I had to go.

I walked through the door physically exhausted, but emotionally high, and told Joanne of all my adventures before finally falling into bed for some much needed rest.

Later in the afternoon Rebecca and James arrived home from school. I had just woken up and had my first hot shower in days. James wanted to jump all over me, but Rebecca was less interested nowadays. She had hit the terrible teens a few months earlier, and the daughter who had once adored me, barely spoke more than a mumble to me now.

"Have you missed me, Bex," I said as I saw her. "Yes," she said as she walked in the room, before leaving just as quickly to put on music upstairs. It was difficult being a teenager, that was for sure. They went through so many changes both physically and emotionally, that they didn't know themselves half the time. But it was hard being a father too, watching your child grow up as you aged yourself - and in truth, I was beginning to feel old.

James on the other hand gave me too much attention and wanted to make up for lost time as he started to play fight with me. "Give your dad time to recover," Joanne shouted, as he pummeled me whilst I sat on the couch.

"Get off a minute," I said "There's some breaking news on the TV and I want to find out what's been happening while I've been away." He jumped on my knee facing me eye-to-eye, waving his fist menacingly in the air. "Oh something will be breaking in a minute," he said, giggling "and it won't be the news."

And with that I was brought back to earth with a thump…

Message from Afar

It took me a few days to recover my strength, but as it returned I knew I had an important message to deliver.

Edward had given me his sister's address and asked that I contact her for him and tell her he was safe and well. It was an awkward duty which had befallen me in a way, because I was about to knock on the door of a complete stranger and give her a profound message from someone she hadn't heard from for a very long time. But meeting Edward had happened in such bizarre circumstances, I couldn't ignore its importance.

I drove the short distance to the lady's house and pulled up, still unsure how to introduce myself. I knocked on the door and waited for a moment, before an elderly figure approached slowly from within the house aided by a Zimmer frame.

"Hello," I said as she opened the door. "You don't know me," I said with a smile to disguise my unease, "but I have a message for you from your brother Edward whom I met in Zululand last week." "Hello," she said, without showing the surprise I had been anticipating. "Edward gave me your address and asked that I pop by and tell you that he's safe and well in Zimbabwe." Edward's sister was elderly herself, and in poor health, yet she didn't seemed to find the message as strange as I did, but instead received it warmly with a smile of understanding, which I found quite odd. It was a cold day and as I continued to talk I could see my breath with each word I spoke. It wasn't long before I had delivered my message, and didn't want to hang around too long, still feeling a little uncomfortable with the whole situation.

As I finished relaying Edward's message his sister smiled again and thanked me for coming to her with the news.

"OK then, I'll be off," I said shyly, as the neighbour who had been in his garden eavesdropping, turned away so as not to stare at me as I walked back up the path. I climbed into my car, and decided not to dwell on what had happened – I had played my part, and that was all that I could do.

I returned home and needed to take Joanne shopping. The holidays were approaching and in truth it had been a long, hard year for us both and I was looking forward to seeing its end and starting anew in 2008.

And as usual I had no clue as to what was about to happen…

The World's Gone Mad

Last year friends had been helping me form a charity called Banana Appeal, with a mission to expand the schemes I had set up. Banana Appeal was granted charitable status in January 2008, and I should have been full of energy. But deep inside me something was very wrong, and by the time I realised what it was, it was too late...

As the months rolled by, wars raged across the planet, blighting the lives of millions. The U.K. and U.S. were still fighting in Iraq and Afghanistan and death and destruction was never far from the news. Gaza was under siege from Israel, leaving mothers and children to starve and suffer inhumanely, as a battle of religions was played out in the *holy lands*. Tibet continued to be suppressed by the Chinese and tensions rose to boiling point as the Beijing Olympics approached.

The Sudanese government continued to persecute, murder and displace its own people in Darfur; whilst Africa as a whole suffered from countless unreported droughts, famines and wars, compounded by poverty, corruption and global inaction.

Russia and Georgia went to war, as more scenes of horror hit the headlines, and the world seemed on the brink of nuclear meltdown as America pushed ahead with its controversial plans of a missile defence site in Poland, something which the Russians would never allow in their backyard.

Climate change, global warming and deforestation continued at an unstoppable pace, threatening our very existence, whilst we continued to churn out gas guzzling 4x4's and flatten ancient forests relentlessly in the name of economic prosperity.

Glaciers were melting and sea levels rising; weather patterns were changing, and natural disasters were escalating. Around the world wildfires raged from Australia to Greece, Athens to California, whilst floods and mudslides washed away countless communities on every continent.

Storms, hurricanes, typhoons and cyclones battered country after country, bringing death and destruction in their wake.

The world's resources were diminishing and demand was growing. The world's population was growing by quarter of a million people a day and the Earth could no longer keep pace with the unsustainable consumption of its resources in our capitalist economy, driven by money, greed and power.

Poverty, hunger, pandemics and preventable diseases killed millions with each passing month, whilst political and corporate fraud raged rampant.

Man's actions were causing death and disaster on a global scale in front of my eyes and if I ever lost my mind to madness, then I certainly wasn't alone.

At the same time I was trying to feed 1,500 children a day, and struggling badly, and I slowly slipped into a deep depression which lasted for months...

Awakening

I hadn't realised the dreadful effects of depression before but luckily, I quickly began to regain my senses.

It was a difficult time for me; especially as I was someone who had been so positive and energetic in the past, then to suddenly find myself weak and vulnerable, depressed and defeated.

A year ago I had been as fit as anyone I knew, jumping around in full-on karate classes and doing hundreds of sits-ups each day, performing flying kicking through blocks of wood or knocking around 18-stone punch bags for fun. Then all of a sudden I could barely summon the energy to move...

They say every cloud has a silver lining, and from these depressing days I learnt much about myself and about others. I'd always been a fighter and had often wondered why the Zulu seemed so resigned to their fate and not fought hard to beat it – but it was only through my own weakness that could I begin to appreciate theirs.

I realised there was a communal depression flowing through Zululand; a debilitating depression caused by poverty and a sense of absolute hopelessness – and it was as deadly as any pandemic.

This communal depression seemed almost contagious too, spreading from person to person, slowly sapping the life from the whole community as it did.

I knew then, that the only way to defeat this depression was to empower the people and bring them some hope.

Banana Appeal was struggling to feed 1,500 children a day – and in all honesty I didn't know how much longer I could keep feeding them.

The charity, Just One Child, had been helping me operate the fruit to school schemes though part of 2007, whilst friends had been setting up our own charity.

Banana Appeal took over the feeding schemes from February, with the aim to boost the number of children we were feeding in order to provide a million school meals a year.

But by June we had all but failed through lack of fundraising, and most of the promises of help I had received previously from people, had evaporated into thin air.

This included Father Ned who had never returned my calls or followed up on his promise of help and fundraising.

In the end I stop calling him, and the next time I saw him was in the newspapers, smiling and famous as the local Merseyside priest who had conducted Wayne Rooney's lavish £5 million marriage to Coleen McLoughlin in Italy!

"What a crazy messed up world we live in," I said to Joanne as I read of Father Ned in disbelief. "You've done all you can and you have to ignore what other people do," Joanne said with a sympathetic smile as she tried to perk me up.

Luckily, whilst I had been in the throes of my mini mid-life crisis, my story had been on a journey of its own, travelling the world and telling of the Zulu children's plight.

Just as Banana Appeal was about to run out of money, a man who had heard of my work via social networking organised a charity firewalk, raising enough money to feed over a hundred thousand school meals of fruit!

A month later, another man who I had connected with through social networking, organised a charity 'death march' in his home country of Belgium. He and others attempted to walk 100 kilometres in 24-hours and succeeded in raising enough money to feed a hundred and fifty thousand school meals of fruit!

Combined, they helped feed over a quarter of a million meals of fruit and saved the charity from the brink of collapse.

I knew from my emails that word of my work had travelled across the UK and to the U.S, France, Holland, Belgium, Germany and around the world through social networking. Some people sent donations, others kind words of support, others sent children's toys, clothes or books.

Then a few weeks later, my story somehow found its way home, back to Africa and into the hands of the Zululand press.

I received an excited email from the editor of the paper telling me he couldn't believe what I was doing in his country and how he wanted to get his whole community behind my projects!

He was incredibly well connected and had many contacts within the large mineral and mining corporates in Richards Bay. He regularly interviewed top politicians too and wanted to arrange a meeting for me with the ANC leader Jacob Zuma.

His email explained Jacob Zuma may support my work, because by an incredible twist of fate, he had been born and raised in the very town where I had fed so many children - Nkandla!

The editor was going away for a month but wanted to meet with me in Africa on his return.

I couldn't believe it! After all this time I finally felt I had the break I had needed for so very long for.

Tsunami

I started to plan a return trip to Zululand to meet the press who were going to introduce me to a number of top executives within some of South Africa's largest corporations.

The potential of this could be enormous for the children we were feeding, and I was struggling to contain my excitement.

The FIFA World Cup was being hosted by South Africa in 2010 and big business would make great efforts to prove their social responsibility, as a billion people turned to watch football in their country.

Better still, I had a good chance of meeting ANC leader Jacob Zuma, who may use his influence to support my work, or even promote my simple feeding schemes further afield across South Africa!

But a storm had been brewing for well over a year now; a financial storm which was about to wipe out banks, businesses, stock markets, jobs, economies and countries.

Reckless lending by greedy bankers and the collapse of the sub-prime mortgage market in the U.S., had been causing problems for some time now.

Britain had already experienced the effects of this the previous year, after depositors of Northern Rock withdrew £1bn in a day, on a run on the bank, resulting in it later being nationalised.

A month after Northern Rock had been rescued, Wall Street's fifth largest bank, Bear Stearns suffered a similar fate, as it lost 98% of its value and came to the brink of insolvency, before being taken over by another bank with government backing.

The International Monetary Fund had already warned losses from the credit crunch could exceed $1 trillion, as the effects from sub-prime mortgage lending spread to other sectors, including property, consumer credit and company debt.

This had only been the beginning though, and within weeks of my invitation to travel back to Zululand to met corporate supporters for my work, the US government had to step in to rescue America's two largest lenders, Fannie Mae and Freddie Mac, who combined owned outstanding mortgages in the US, amounting to more than $5 trillion.

A little over a week later, and America giants Lehman Brothers went bust as Merrill Lynch had to be taken over by the Bank of America, and the US Federal Reserve was forced to announce an $85 billion rescue package for another ailing American giant, AIG. Defining moments in history and the start of a global 'credit crunch'.

Not long after this and the U.S. Congress was forced to make a $700 billion bail out package for the American financial system, in the biggest intervention in the markets since the Great Depression of the 1930's!

Some economists believed that this, along with the cost of ongoing wars in Iraq and Afghanistan, could send the U.S. national debt level beyond $11 trillion dollars.

To put this into perspective, America's entire gold reserves were about $200 billion, meaning the country was drowning in debt which it could never repay.

On a bank note are the words 'the bank promises to pay the bearer' and this promise used to be known as the gold standard i.e. that the national bank held gold reserves equal to the amount of money in circulation and could therefore honour the value of the note. The gold standard had been scrapped during the first and second world wars – but today the promise was worthless – there wasn't enough gold in the world to cover national debt of countries like the U.S. and they weren't alone.

Some people even speculated the only way the U.S. could clear this debt was to collapse the dollar completely and replace it with a North American union currency, similar to the Euro, the Amero. This would press the reset button on America's debt, but the dollar would become worthless overnight and the impact globally was too terrifying to even think about…

Whatever was to happen next the free market had failed, and as the world stood on the precipice of a devastating global recession, my chances of securing any kind of financial support from major corporates in South Africa had evaporated before my eyes.

In the coming months the world continued to implode as a financial tsunami swept across the globe, wiping out financial giants that had stood strong through world wars and great depressions.

But whilst this historical event was unfolding, two black politicians were making history themselves, as they battled to become the most powerful men on earth.

By November history had been made in the U.S. as Barack Obama won the elections to become the first black president of America.

Meanwhile in Africa, Jacob Zuma had just ousted his rival, South African president Mbeki – paving the way for him to become the most powerful man in Africa at the next elections, which were only months away.

The Circle of Life

As the year came to an end a deep recession was underway. I was physically and financially drained from stress at work and worrying about the feeding schemes, and as Christmas came and went, we like many recession hit families, had to tighten our belts.

As 2009 began I was still struggling to feed 1,500 children a day. We'd provided 300,000 school meals last year, but the going was tough. I started my journey as a sprint, to find and help a desperate child, but my race had somehow turned into a marathon; an endless marathon that seemed to have no finishing line.

Fundraising events had been few and far between, but luckily a lady called Sonia was holding a large Valentines charity ball in a few weeks and it should bring in some much needed funds.

Sonia had worked hard arranging the event, and I had agreed to give a short talk on the night, but the recession was making it next to impossible to raise cash. Nevertheless it was a great night and nearly 100 people attended, helping to feed many tens of thousands of children.

But we were supplying 30,000 meals a month and despite the success of the night the charity was struggling - and I wasn't sure how much longer I could keep up the schemes.

I was still in contact with Sister Hedwig by email and we sent each other personal messages often. Her sister was sick with AIDS and

I sent her a little money whenever I could and had managed to send some just before Christmas. A few days after the charity ball, I received an email from Hedwig.

email from Africa.......

Dear Kevin...

.....Life is hard here in South Africa Kevin because of this killer disease, I pray day and night that a cure could be found sooner before my sister goes as well. But she feels very strong and happy Kevin you just can not believe what change has happened to this woman. When I went home I gave R900 from that money for food, you know what it does to hold money in your hands when you have not even a cent...These are her cures, and the sugar cane she has been able to plant has added to her happiness... Do you know that Mbali passed her matric and Sne is going from grade 6 this year and Mbali has a baby boy....

"Joanne!" I shouted in shock. "Hedwig says Mbali has had a baby!"

"Crumbs, she's only a young teenager, isn't she," Joanne said, knowing what fate awaited Mbali's child. As Hedwig's message sank in I knew I had to do something for Mbali and her newborn baby.

I knew I had to return to Africa.

A couple of weeks later I was back in Zululand starting another mind blowing journey... and this time I wasn't alone.

The World is Yours

It was early morning as the plane touched down in Johannesburg with a heavy thud, waking me from my world of reminiscing.

I disembarked to the dazzling brightness of the sun, enjoying its warming rays as they touched my skin. The Zululand press had arranged to interview me and they were trying to set up a meeting for me to meet Jacob Zuma to gain his support for my work.

He was in the middle of the presidential elections and was about to become the most powerful man in Africa and campaigning was in full swing. As I went for the connecting flight to Durban I realised I had no idea what magical adventures would transpire over the coming week.

Wow, I thought, I would never know the full consequences of my actions; only that the smallest act continued to ripple outwards, creating an ever-growing wave of hope for the forgotten children of Zululand, as support for their plight started to grow.

I imagined the tragedy if I had never taken that first leap of faith to look for Sne those few short years ago. If I hadn't broken my inhibitions, if I hadn't kept struggling forward when all seemed lost.

My life had been enriched by my enlightening experiences, and I smiled widely, knowing my incredible journey was just about to continue – whilst someone else's could be just about to begin...

When powerful governments, giant corporations, religious groups or large charities act inappropriately, or fail to act at all, it's left to individuals to unite and take action.

All it takes to change the world is the smallest act of kindness.

All it takes to change the world is YOU....

A personal message from Kevin

Thank you for buying this book and I hope you found it inspirational.

Since my first journey in 2005 I've fed over a million school meals of fresh fruit to hungry children. Today, I continue to feed thousands more meals each day, and am laying the foundations to plant 2.5 million fruit trees a year to show how all hungry children in third world communities can be fed through school.

This is only possible because the royalties from each book sold help me feed a child for a month and plant a tree in Africa.

Join me on the next step of my journey

This book may be coming to an end, but the story must continue, and I need your help to write the next chapter.

Please help me create a Guinness World Record by creating the world's first chain book which will feed tens of millions of school meals to desperate children.

Be amazing today

Help me spread word of the plight of the Zulus AND help me make this book a 'chain book' by buying another three copies and gifting them to friends, family, colleagues, school libraries or complete strangers. This will create a magical ripple which will mean each book sold will lead to three more being bought.

Remember, each book you gift will not only feed a child for a month and plant a tree, but also create an ongoing chain reaction, transforming the lives of many.

Please help me save the children and buy three more copies of this book today.

Kevin 'Banana Man' Allen

You can buy further copies of this book online at:

www.ecademy-press.com
www.amazon.com
www.barnesandnoble.com
www.waterstones.com

You can order a copy of this book at any bookstore or by mail order by sending your name and address with a cheque for £14.99 per book + £1.95 postage and packing to:

Banana Appeal
12 Maritime House
Off Alfred's Road
Wirral CH43 5RE

For photographs of the children and for updates please visit our banana blog at Bananaappeal.org

Banana Appeal

Please send to:
Banana Appeal, Office 12, Maritime House, Off Alfreds Road, Wirral CH43 5RE

To :The Manager,

Bank: ....

Bank Address: ....

.... Postcode.................................

Please set up the following Standing Order and debit my/our account accordingly

1. Account details

Account Name: ....

Acc No: ☐ ☐ ☐ ☐ ☐ ☐ ☐ ☐

Account Holding Branch: ....

Sort Code: ☐ ☐ / ☐ ☐ / ☐ ☐

2. Payee details

Organisation you are paying: **Banana Appeal**

Payment reference:

BANANAS ☐ ☐ ☐ ☐ ☐ ☐ ☐ ☐ ☐ ☐ ☐ ☐ ☐ ☐

If you wish, add your name to the reference

Sort Code: **60-17-21**

Account number: **88910326**

3. About the Payment

Frequency of payment:

Monthly: ☐ Quarterly: ☐ Half Yearly: ☐ Yearly: ☐

Date and amount of first payment:

☐☐ / ☐☐ / ☐☐ £ ☐ , ☐☐☐ . ☐☐

Date and amount of ongoing payments:

☐☐ / ☐☐ / ☐☐ £ ☐ , ☐☐☐ . ☐☐

Choose one of the following two option:

1. Date and amount of final payment:

☐☐ / ☐☐ / ☐☐ £ ☐ , ☐☐☐ . ☐☐

2. Until further notice:

☐ (payments made will be made until you cancel this instruction)

4. Confirmation

Signature/s: ....

....

Date: ....

4. Gift Aid Decleration

I / We, ...

of address ....

....

Confirmation that this/these is/are gift aid donation/s to Banana Appeal and that I/we have/will have paid sufficient UK tax to cover the tax that Banana Appeal will reclaim.

Signature/s ....

....

Date: ....

Lightning Source UK Ltd.
Milton Keynes UK
02 February 2010

149436UK00001B/3/P